A Violation
Against Women

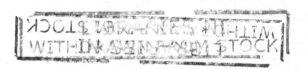
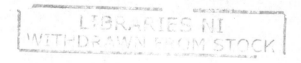

First published in 2015 by
Liberties Press
140 Terenure Road North | Terenure | Dublin 6W
T: +353 (1) 905 6072 | W: libertiespress.com | E: info@libertiespress.com

Trade enquiries to Gill & Macmillan Distribution
Hume Avenue | Park West | Dublin 12
T: +353 (1) 500 9534 | F: +353 (1) 500 9595 | E: sales@gillmacmillan.ie

Distributed in the United Kingdom by
Turnaround Publisher Services
Unit 3 | Olympia Trading Estate | Coburg Road | London N22 6TZ
T: +44 (0) 20 8829 3000 | E: orders@turnaround-uk.com

Distributed in the United States by
Casemate-IPM | 1950 Lawrence Road | Havertown, PA 19083
T: +1 (703) 661-1586 | E: casemate@casematepublishers.com

ISBN: 978-1-90742-12-9
2 4 6 8 10 9 7 5 3 1

A CIP record for this title is available from the British Library.

Cover design by Liberties Press
Internal design by Liberties Press

A Violation
Against Women

Kathleen Ward

Contents

Introduction

I could have written this book and then kept it locked away in a safe place for a very long time – indeed, forever. Instead, many of my thoughts, and vivid recollections of the event, and much of the writing that I have penned over the last twenty years, I now choose to publish, for several reasons and a variety of people. As writing this book has enhanced my personal healing, it is my greatest hope that it will in some way help *you* too to begin to restore your health if you have been in a similar situation at any time during your life. Your experiences may have been recent or in the more distant past, but that does not matter: it is never too late to heal. Healing does not have set time limits. You must first restore your health before you can move on with your life.

The first reason I am publishing this book is that, perhaps selfishly, I am seeking personal closure following the trauma I endured in 1995 as a result of the reckless, negligent and possibly premeditated behaviour of Dr Michael Neary, obstetrician at Our Lady of Lourdes Hospital in Drogheda, and the system that prevailed in that era. Indeed, it is the same reckless negligence which appears to have spanned a quarter of a century in total, with many women affected at his hands. My trauma occurred during the delivery of my baby by caesarean section on 10 July 1995. I went into the Lourdes Hospital knowing, in advance, that my baby would be delivered by elective caesarean section, but with no idea of the horrendous consequences that lay in store for me and my family.

In writing this book I wish to highlight the many closed doors I encountered over my twenty-year search for answers, and continuous quest for justice. There was a mentality of not rocking the boat, and not questioning doctors.

I was betrayed by the Irish government and the ministers for health at that time – Micheál Martin and, later, Mary Harney – in the narrow, mindless and exclusive way in which they set up the Patient Redress Board following numerous inquiries all those years later.

I want to make public the approach adopted by the reviewing consultants to whom I was referred. It is said that 'the written word lasts forever', and this was certainly the belief system that I encountered in reviewing my files. Medical insensitivity to my experience was at times personally degrading; their belief in the written word in the hospital charts – which they treated as gospel and to which only they were privy – was, during the many subsequent inquiries, often found to be misplaced. Believing the 'written word' – which they may have known was flawed – may have even been their way of excercising medical privilege, serving to make the patient feel insignificant. Thankfully, patients today are much more clued in to their health, far more so than in the last century, when these crimes took place. With the advent of the Internet, people are also constantly researching their conditions and taking less for granted.

Secondly, and perhaps more importantly, I am publishing this book for other women. I know of many women who have stated that they have undergone unplanned hysterectomies (surgical womb removals) at the Lourdes Hospital. Some had only recently been married, and had had their opportunity to conceive and give birth surgically taken away from them, without their knowledge. This procedure was carried out without their control or consent, and performed by means of hysterectomy or oophorectomy (removal of ovaries). Some women only learnt of their fate much later on, in their review appointment.

For others, the surgery was performed during the delivery of their first baby, or during their subsequent deliveries. In some cases, those babies died at birth, or shortly afterwards. But whether it was their first baby or not, nobody had given this man the right to decide on their parity. I wonder if Dr Neary had thought through how his actions would mould the lives of these women and their families? Does he have any idea of the grief he has caused so many families? Does he care?

Many of these women have never been heard of in the public domain following their trauma, either by choice or opportunity. This does not mean they have not suffered, nor indeed that they may not still suffer. Many felt bullied into silence by family or medical professionals, who either made them feel stupidly inarticulate or that the procedure was a genuinely life-saving surgery. Some even felt personal shame as a result of their outcome. Whatever our background, many of us will carry this hurt to our graves.

The purpose of this book is to encourage women who have suffered injustice never to give up in their quest for truth and justice. It is dedicated to women who have suffered similar experiences to me, and may remain isolated in silence; those who have chosen not to speak out about their tragedy; and those who have felt unable to speak out about their experience.

This book is also written for men who have a wife, partner, sister, mother or friend who has endured a similar fate at the hands of Dr Neary or other medical professionals while under their care, and men who have themselves encountered difficult experiences or unwarranted surgeries at the hands of the medical profession.

Thirdly, I have written this book for the many excellent doctors, nurses and others in the caring profession. Most of these amazing professionals never receive praise and thanks for the outstanding work they do on a daily basis. Many of these doctors, nurses and other medical professionals feel deeply tainted and distrusted by the public following the inquiry reports in the wake of the Neary revelations. This, in itself, is an injustice to those hard-working individuals.

To those working in the medical profession:

- Never be afraid to speak up in the cause of right.

- Remember the Hippocratic oath, 'First do no harm'. 'Harm' extends beyond the physical impact to the very language used when relating to patients. Is your message always relayed with understanding, compassion and competency, or is it controlled by dominance, self-glorification, self-gratification or fear?

- Do not be afraid to be a whistleblower if you see or feel that wrong is being done: everyone has a moral obligation to relay the truth.

- Always bear in mind that a human being has physical, mental, emotional and spiritual components in their make-up. Each component is of equal importance, though not always equally addressed in medical circles. Allopathic medicine usually concentrates more on physical signs and symptoms, often omitting the emotional consequences of a condition.

This book is written to highlight how your mental health can be destroyed by unprecedented actions and inappropriate treatment by others, including those in the medical profession. This can happen following a misguided or split-second decision, one with long-lasting repercussions.

Depression is the impression left by fear. Serious mental-health disruption knows no boundaries, crosses all barriers, creeds and classes and can have unpredictable adverse effects. There are no hard and fast rules on how soon after the event this may occur, or how long it may last. For many, it can become a never-ending nightmare: a horror movie in which many of the scenes are replayed time and time again; and from which there may be no awakening. It can be like being tortured by some unknown force. Nobody is immune to this disruption during their lifetime. Yet it is the one area of healthcare most hidden from society. No one chooses illness from the menu of life, but each one of us is vulnerable, and can tumble at any time. We can all get lost in the fog that shrouds our life, since life is an imperfect journey.

I wish to clarify that I am in no way anti-doctor or anti-allopathic medicine. I know many wonderful doctors and nurses who enter their professions to devote their lives to the cause of excellent care and the cause of what is right for their patients – to make a real difference. Many go beyond the call of duty.

I am a nurse, midwife, antenatal teacher and herbalist, who

has been trained to deliver a duty of care to those in need at all times. My training taught me that without patients, I was not needed. It ingrained in me the importance of treating every human being with whom I came into contact with respect, dignity and honesty. I was taught that it was an honour and a privilege to serve the sick. This approach, sadly, was not what I experienced in 1995, nor in the years that followed.

This book is a sincere thank-you to those who journeyed with me on my quest for wellness, including my family, friends and therapists. As Jack Canfield once said: 'Everything you want is on the other side of fear.'

I have been encouraged to write this book, and to outline my personal experience, by a cross-section of people. In 1995, I endured a deeply flawed duty of care from Dr Neary, Our Lady of Lourdes Hospital, the North-Eastern Health Board and the minister for health. Not only did I not receive the treatment I was entitled to and privately paying for – the treatment that I needed and deserved – but, following the assault, abuse and neglect that I suffered, there has been a major cover-up. I do not believe that anything has really changed, despite all the declarations of 'This must never be allowed to happen again.' There appears to be more firefighting of scandals than implementation of recommendations.

I still want to know the truth of what happened to me, and why. To err is human; to cover up is deceit. Those who kept their silence or chose to turn a blind eye for all those years are, in my view, complicit in the crimes Neary committed.

Of course, I expect detractors, but each will have to look first to their own conscience and personal agenda. Why are staff still protecting Neary's actions, and why have they maintained their silence, knowing that all was not well with his practices?

What you have before you is an honest account of my experience and the ensuing inquiries.

Chapter 1
Who Am I to Speak?

I am an ordinary Irish woman, born in the late 1950s in the quiet and very beautiful seaside resort of Ballyheigue, in north Kerry. This village is noted for its six-mile beach, which stretches on to Banna strand. Some famous residents have lived and visited over the years. This is where author Christy Brown, author of *My Left Foot*, lived out his final days. It is currently home to famed local authors of parish history, namely Micheal O Halloran and Brian McMahon. It is home to my nephew, author Aidan Lucid, whose writing is taking him to greater heights, further afield in Los Angeles. In more recent times, this is also the village where internationally renowned fashion designer Don O'Neill was born and reared.

I was not born with a silver spoon in my mouth: I was fortunate to be born into a poor family. I say 'fortunate' as, though life was very poor and very, very simple, everything we got we appreciated, and worked really hard for. For all of my life this start has kept me firmly grounded, never forgetting my humble beginnings, and above all never forgetting where I came from. It has helped me remain humble and compassionate, to respect the feelings of others and appreciate everything I have, upholding honesty as the best policy, all in the name of God, as was the teaching I was reared with.

We moved from my grandmother's farmhouse to our own home when I was four, to a simple council cottage built on one acre of land, which my parents purchased from a nearby farmer. But encased in that house was a lot of love from and sacrifice on the part of my parents; they turned it from a house into a home. In those days, we would have been known as 'cottiers', since the house was provided by the county council on our own land.

At first, we had one light bulb that was moved from room to room as required. Pennies were scarce, and each one was a prisoner. Expenditure was well thought out before it was made. Dad was a labourer and carpenter, and earned little money – there was not much work and wages were low. He co-owned a threshing machine with my uncle, which they would work together in the harvest season, going from farm to farm within our parish and neighbouring parishes. He later worked with a German baroness, who had come to our parish and set up a cottage industry. It gave much-needed employment. Dad made sugán chairs and other crafts, which the baroness sold locally or exported. Mam helped milk a neighbouring farmer's cows in return for a free gallon of milk daily. She also knitted men's sweaters for the German cottage industry. There were two main styles, Aran and fisherman's rib. I made 'Irish cottages' using matchboxes and scrap material, receiving one penny for each house delivered. Life was hard but we children were very happy in our world; it was all we knew and we enjoyed it. We made our own fun, as toys were few. We thought everybody lived like this.

Of course, as youngsters we had no idea how our parents 'went without' to feed us: Mam used to drink black tea to save the milk for us as children, and dinners were simple, mostly consisting of mashed potatoes (called 'pandy') mixed with fried bacon bits saved from the curing of their own pig. Any vegetables we ate were grown in our garden. Our parents were very religious, God-fearing people. We were taught never to pass a Church without 'saying "Hello" to God'. The rosary and 'the trimmings' were very important parts of daily life. My older brother and I would play marbles under the chairs when we got bored during the interminable prayer time, much to the dismay of my parents. The nearby Our Lady's Well was a frequent and famous place of pilgrimage in my youth, especially on sunny Sundays when we headed to the local beach; the grotto had to be visited first. To this day, that place holds special favour both in the parish and beyond, with the diocesan bishop concelebrating Mass annually on 8 September. It was called The Pattern Day.

I remember when my elder brother was asked to be an altar server: my parents had to pay five shillings for his surplice and soutane. This involved lengthy discussion around the turf fire, as all the money my parents had at the time was five shillings: but they gave it in the name of God. The next day, a letter arrived from Mam's aunt in New Jersey. It contained $40, an unheard of sum in those days. The letter was tattered and torn, but the dollars remained within: an indication of the honesty that was prevalent at that time. Mam taught us that this was God's way of repaying them for the sacrifice they had made. This was the environment in which we were raised. I was clothed in hand-me-downs from a wealthier neighbour's child, and infrequent parcels from mother's aunt in New Jersey. This included my First Communion dress. I thought this was great – it seemed as if I had lots of new clothes.

I was the second of three living children. Another sibling had been stillborn a couple of years before the birth of my youngest brother, my junior by seven years. In those days we were not told what was happening, but I remember my dad taking the stillborn baby on his bike to be buried, wrapped in a white sheet. It was never spoken about afterwards, but how difficult that must have been for Mam and Dad. There was no counselling for them back then. In later years, I learned that the baby had to be buried outside my paternal family's tomb, on unconsecrated land, as the baby had not been baptised. Such is the cruelty of man-made rules that existed within our church.

My elder brother and I were the very best buddies as we were close in age, he being two years older. We did the daily walk to school together, and participated in many talent contests and school concerts as singers, with my brother playing the guitar. He was self-taught, and sure, we thought we were great entertainers. These opportunities were important to us as children. My brother went on to launch his own band as his livelihood, and I undertook some voice training when I moved to Dublin.

Primary school is a very mixed bag of memories, mostly negative ones. I went to the local two-teacher school aged four, as I could read and write and was exempted from senior infants. I went straight into first class. We had to keep our lunch on our knees, as rats ran freely through the classroom. School life was difficult, as teachers were hard on students. This was probably the order of the day at the time: corporal punishment was allowed. While that still did not make it right to beat children incessantly, they beat the thrash out of us on a daily basis. The teacher that I had in first class used to lift me by my hair and swing me around. It was probably because of this that my hair fell out in clumps, and I had to be treated by a doctor. No questions were ever asked as to why this had happened, nor any attempt made to seek out if this was abuse. In those days we did not dare tell this at home, as our parents would have thought that we had done something wrong to deserve it. Fear was a big part of every school day, with daily, humiliating reminders of the fact that we were poor. One such episode was when my parents did not have the money for me to go on the school tour to Dublin. I did not really understand what all that meant back then – I was just a child. Of course, we now know, with the benefit of psychological research, that this sort of treatment in one's childhood, especially before the age of seven, plays a huge part in our well-being as we get older.

I regret not having a sister, but one of my wonderful long-time sisters-in-law fills that space very well. My younger brother was only nine years old when I left home to begin work in Dublin, so I did not have an opportunity to get to know him as well as my elder brother.

I went out to work on Saturdays as a cleaner in the local presbytery. I was ten. That was both great and scary. It was great in that I got paid, which made me feel good, as I could contribute to the family income, but it was also terrifying, as the housekeeper always seemed cross. The next summer, when I was eleven years old, I went to work for the local German baroness. I was the childminder to her grandchildren when they came to visit from France and Germany. This was enjoyable, though not very remunerative. My summer holidays were afterwards spent working in a local business, which comprised a shop, a restaurant and tourist accommodation. This too was great, though we worked hard for seven days a week and twelve hours a day, earning £3 per week. I happily cycled off to work every morning at 7 AM. I met some different and lovely people there. In my childish innocence I thought the people who went on holidays 'must be loaded'. I had no idea what 'holidays' actually meant, as we did not have any. More importantly for me, my £3 subsidised home life, and gained me greater confidence.

Interspersed with this, Dad grew a couple of acres of sugar-beet on conacre or, as it was called locally, 'scor'. My brother and I hated it, as we would be sent out to hoe and weed the seemingly endless acres every summer. Going to the bog for turf-cutting was much more fun, as we would get a ride on my grandfather's donkey.

My maternal grandmother was my idol and protector. We lived with her until I was four, and I was her only grand-daughter at the time. In my memory, she was a kind and very talented lady. Nan lived on a farm, but was also a wonderful seamstress, making bed quilts, altar cloths, lace and other crafts, using her Singer sewing machine. She often came to visit after we moved house, and would stay for a few weeks at a time: we hated it when she went home. As a little girl I loved fixing her long silver hair into a bun and helping her with little personal duties. She usually dressed in navy or black, as she was long widowed. She wore a black shawl to Mass, and would always have Silvermints in her pocket. We loved it when she sat beside us, as we were sure of getting a Silvermint. She did not enjoy great health, and walked with a limp. Nan always said to me: 'You will make a great nurse one day. Be sure and look after old people.' Since we lived a distance from my paternal grandparents, visits were infrequent but always enjoyable, as there was a large extended household living there. Fatefully, I did become a nurse, and worked in a geriatric hospital for fifteen years. Nan sadly died in her eighties when I was a first-year student nurse, so she never lived to see her dream come true. However, I feel sure she knew from that better place she's gone to; I hope I lived out the dream she had for me, and made her proud. Her death proved to be a terribly hard time for me, and something I did not come to terms with for several years. There was a family decision made, in conjunction with the parish priest, not to relay the news of her sudden death to me as I was in the middle of my nursing exams: they feared it would affect my academic performance. When I came home the following week, not only did I learn that she was dead, but that she had also already been buried. I never got to say my goodbyes to my nan, a source of great personal regret.

I sat my Leaving Certificate aged sixteen, after which I became very ill and ended up in hospital for three months. I had my appendix removed, but was subsequently found to be anaemic. Treatment for anaemia then was different to today, and it meant that I was hospitalised for that entire summer while they got my iron stores raised to normal.

In September 1973 I left home to begin work as a civil servant in Dublin, at the Department of Posts & Telegraphs in Townsend Street. I was excited but sad, and fearful, as I was not very worldly. I had never travelled far from my home or even stayed away from it for a single night. Dublin sounded like a distant and scary place. It seemed almost as far away as America. My dad accompanied me on that train journey to Dublin to help me find accommodation. As we parted ways on O'Connell Bridge I was sure he was going to give me some advice. Instead, he simply said: 'Kathleen, never forget your prayers.' That spoke volumes to me, and as I got older that advice has had a lasting impression. It has served me well throughout my life, especially during my later years of enforced health difficulties.

I lived in a six-bed dormitory, several floors up, in a Mountjoy Square hostel for girls, run by the Sisters of Charity. I stayed there for a year. While the sisters were very kind, it was not always a pleasant place as our few worldly possessions often got robbed, presumably by other residents. It would be lonely there at the weekends as most of the other girls went home, but I could not afford this luxury. Staying there did at least enable me to save £16 weekly from my wages, for my nurse training fee of £166. If I was to progress to be a nurse I knew I had to earn the fee, otherwise I could not go. I had by now been accepted for general nurse training at Our Lady of Lourdes Hospital, commencing March 1975. At the same time I would send £5 home most weeks: this was badly needed, as there was still my younger brother to fend for and send to school.

That is what my generation did: those who had work shared their income with their families at home. I call us 'the trapped generation'. We, the offspring, sent money home to our parents; now, as parents ourselves, we send money to our kids because of the recessionary times in which we live.

I vividly remember the day of the Dublin bombing. I was to collect a sweater for my brother in Guiney's on Abbey Street, but forgot the money, so I went back to the hostel. I was at the front door when the bomb went off just down the street, causing death and devastation. Of course, Guiney's was one of the places most severely damaged, and many lost their lives there. Little did I know then that I would end up living in Monaghan one day, where bombs had gone off on that same day.

In March 1995 I went to the Lourdes Hospital, Drogheda, County Louth, to commence my training in general nursing. My parents could not afford to accompany me on my initiation as they did not have the fare to travel from Kerry. So my cousin, Father Tom O'Connor, a priest in the order of St Camillus who lived in Dublin, was summoned to make the journey with me. I found that a very tough start, as most other girls were there with their families, but I was resilient and determined. The students' parents were taken in to meet the sisters, but as I did not have my parents there Father Tom and I were asked to wait out in the foyer. Trepidation reigned as I knew nobody, but Father Tom was very reassuring. Over my time there I made many lifelong friendships.

This hospital was set up by Mother Mary Martin, founder of the Medical Missionaries of Mary order of nuns, in 1933. Training was strict, fair and mostly wonderful. Of course, there were times when I found it so tough that I thought, *I want out of here*, but as student colleagues we helped each other through such times – going home without a job was not an option. In those days we worked on the wards after an initial three-month 'block/in school' period called 'PTS' (preliminary training session). If we did not pass our exams, we ran the risk of being turfed out. We studied on days off and most evenings after work. In 1978 I graduated as a general nurse. I moved back to Tralee to work at St Catherine's Hospital that summer, on permanent night-duty. This was a wonderful experience as it was busy. I returned to the Lourdes Hospital in October of that year to begin training as a midwife. This was a year-long course which I enjoyed immensely. I graduated in October 1979 knowing that midwifery was my first love.

Meanwhile, I had fallen in love with a Monaghan man and married in October 1979, two weeks after my final examinations. We moved to Monaghan to live. Peter was a busy shop owner: he sold carpets, beds, window blinds and general household goods. I quickly got work in the local geriatric hospital, St Mary's, Castleblayney, commencing on Christmas Eve 1979. In those days, you took work when offered, otherwise you did not get a second chance, such was the abundance of nurses available at the time and the shortage of work opportunities. We were coming out of the recession of the 1980s, but it really meant nothing to me as I had never been fiscally privileged. It felt like, by working in a geriatric hospital, I was fulfilling the ambition my nan had had for me. Life was wonderful then: we hadn't a bob to our name, but that was nothing new. Our new home was very basic, but it was ours. We were happy and had great hopes for the future – since we both had work we hoped we could create a good life. Our many plans for the future included our intention to move back to Kerry in the next couple of years; but to my eternal regret and sadness, and that of my parents, we never did permanently return to Ballyheigue.

Since midwifery was my first love and I was working as a staff nurse in a geriatric hospital due to its proximity, I trained as an antenatal teacher in 1981. I first trained by undertaking an Irish course run by An Bord Altranais in Dublin. I then went to Alston

Hall in Preston, England, to complete further training in the British regime. I taught privately and became renowned locally for my teaching. Things never happen without a reason, they say, and this was true for me. My husband's business suffered serious setbacks at that time, through multiple robberies. Living close to the border, robberies were then common. My teaching skills supplemented our income. My children also loved the class nights as they used to bring the tea, or rather, the biscuits, to the class – and they always managed to polish off the remaining biscuits.

Our first beautiful daughter, Arlene, was born in 1982. She suffered numerous chest infections from an early age, usually ending with antibiotics being prescribed. This quickly led to her developing asthma and requiring lots of inhalers. Her progressive ill health continued in a downward spiral. She was constantly on high doses of medications that made little difference to her condition. When she developed pneumonia her general condition rapidly deteriorated in the most frightening way. It was suggested to me to try reflexology treatment for her recovery. Being medically trained, this suggestion seemed outrageous, as thinking outside the medical model had not been part of my training. After all, she was seeing an expensive private paediatrician on an ongoing basis, and this had to be the only way to go – or so I blindly thought at the time.

But once again the hand of fate beckoned, and when Arlene became more seriously ill at the end of her second year, I decided to try reflexology as a last resort. Allergy testing was included as part of the treatment, and she was quickly cured when certain foods were eliminated. Her therapist encouraged me to undertake the training course and qualify as a reflexologist, even if I were to only use this therapy on the family. The therapy was relatively new, and few people were aware of its existence. My daughter's experience converted me to holistic medicine. I started my training, and began a beautiful new chapter in my life. I'd got the bug – I was eager to learn more and more. On the reflexology course I met someone who encouraged me to study child psychology, which I duly pursued. While studying for that course I met another person who encouraged me to enrol in a nutrition course. As nurses we were taught the basics of nutrition but developed no in-depth knowledge. I went on to undertake many and various nutrition courses over the ensuing years. It may seem as if I was gullible, but I had developed an insatiable taste for knowledge in this field.

I was nursing full-time and did not have as much time to practice my reflexology therapy as I would have liked. I did initially practise on friends and family, though, when I had the opportunity – and subsequently on family referrals, as I wanted, and needed, to earn money to further my studies. Above all, I saw first-hand the difference that this therapy was making in people's lives, and the positive impacts that it was having on their health. Thankfully, I became renowned for the results I was achieving. To help someone improve their health is priceless and rewarding. I had no fancy treatment quarters – I worked from my sitting room, as I had when hosting my antenatal classes.

The ensuing years were interesting – even a little crazy – because of the gruelling schedule that I undertook. My second angelic daughter, Karen, was born in 1984, and my third daughter, Edel, was born in 1986. My precious and only son was born a year later in 1987. I then had four beautiful and healthy kids under the age of six. I was working permanently on nightduty by choice, to curtail childminding costs. Meanwhile, my mother-in-law had come to live with us, as she was frail and incapacitated from years of severe arthritis. Being on night-duty meant that I could look after her personal care, as I did not enjoy having home help.

I was an eternal student, and life was hectic.

★

I miscarried in 1990, which was very emotionally painful, as I blamed myself for having been too over-committed in the early stages of the pregnancy. But God needed an angel, and I had to unwillingly return my baby back to him. In the aftermath, I found that the physical care I received in the hospital wonderful, but the emotional care was non-existent. The best they could do was to say, 'This happens in one in five pregnancies. You have four healthy children, so what are you crying about?' Go home and get on with it, was the attitude.

My mother-in-law passed to her eternal reward at our home early in 1991. We missed her unbelievably, as she had been a huge and beautiful part of our family life for seven years; the children missed her immeasurably but have very fond memories of their frail, gentle grandmother. Our fourth beautiful daughter, Kerrie, was born in September of that year, which was another wonderful blessing. It is strange, but with life being so busy we do not always stop to thank God and appreciate the blessings we have in our lives.

Life was busy but I was very organised; we were a good family team and everybody pitched in with chores. I enjoyed all the fun activities with my kids. My family were (and are) my life. They were all involved in swimming, music, singing and football, which was terrific, but also meant that we acted as permanent taxis. The children learned to cook from an early age, either standing on chairs or sitting on the table, as each took turns in whatever we were making. It usually ended up a total mess, with flour everywhere, but it was such fun. More importantly, they are all now self-sufficient in their culinary skills and very capable cooks.

Christmas was manic in our house. The children all took part in mixing the twenty puddings, from the end of November. I cooked Christmas dinners for those living alone, the aged, St Vincent de Paul – whatever was needed at each particular Christmas. This was a method of teaching my children to give to those who had less, and bring a little joy into others' lives, especially at that time of year. Even though we were struggling financially on many levels it taught the children the real meaning of Christmas. Christmas Eve was organised but busy; the cooking was done early, then my husband would do the deliveries. The kids enjoyed this – they would all climb into the back of the car to accompany Peter, and would be stuffed full of treats as they delivered the goodies.

Christmas Day was equally hectic as all the children took part in the Christmas Day swim at Lough Muckno, Castleblayney, raising money for the African Kitui Missions. Local priests and nuns did mission work there in Africa over those years, so every contribution was welcome to assist them. Despite early Christmas-morning protestations at having to leave their Santa toys, they loved the swim once they reached Lough Muckno. After their dip in the often snow-laden waters they got sweets and soup, which tasted all the more special. Of course, I was on duty for many Christmas Days at the hospital, but we always managed to coordinate all these activities.

The trips to Kerry to visit my parents were special. We would pack all the children into the car for the long journey. Before we were ten miles down the road there would be a chorus of 'Are we there yet?' Except when we attempted to say the rosary and they would all pretend to be asleep; how history repeats itself. They loved visiting their grandparents and going to the nearby beach for slides on the sand dunes, climbing the rocks and splashing around in the water.

Sadly, my dad passed away in 2002 aged eighty, partly from misdiagnosis and mismanagement of his illness in the local hospital. In my experience, there is a serious disregard of the elderly in many general hospitals, especially towards anyone aged seventy-plus. My mother was so heartbroken by his passing that she started to die a little every day after that. They were very close, having been married for almost fifty years; it was as if her right arm had been wrenched from its socket. Mam developed rapid thyroid cancer in 2006 and, despite a prognosis of survival for up to a year, she was dead three weeks later. I had just brought her to our home twelve hours earlier, so that I could care for her. I found her rapid demise very difficult to cope with, and her death changed my relationship with home forever. The house quickly became 'bricks and mortar' and home as I had known it was no more.

I studied child psychology, nutrition, bio-resonance and vega-testing, counselling and many other courses, culminating in a four-year course in herbalism and homeopathy. The entire training spanned a twenty-year period following my graduation from my nursing programme and conversion to holistic medicine. I had to pace my studies as I needed to keep rotating money back into courses, all of which were expensive, with no grant aid available for health businesses. I remember on one occasion going up Collon Hill, in County Louth, at 6 AM on a snowy morning on my way to a course in Dublin. I was slipping as far back in the frost and ice as I was going forward, and wondering what it was all about. But I kept going, such was (and is) my passion for what I do.

I nursed at St Mary's Hospital, Castleblayney, for the next fifteen years until September 1994, the latter part in a job-sharing capacity. Fortunately I had a very accommodating matron, Sister Scholastica, for most of those years. But in 1994 I felt a serious crisis of conscience over the medical care of a patient; what I was experiencing in practice was not marrying with the principles I had been trained for, and I found that I was neither being listened to nor heard. So I approached the new matron, outlined my concerns and asked for a career break. She was sympathetic, and advised that I must live according to my conscience. A career break was granted quite quickly, much to my surprise. That threw me into another flurry: I had five children at that time. My husband was by now mostly unemployed, aside from a small farm holding. I was suddenly no longer in receipt of a monthly cheque from the health board as a nurse. I will never forget the look on Peter's face the day I told him I had quit nursing, even though I had been threatening this for some time.

But I trusted my faith, so I got on with life. I felt that when I did right by what was in my soul, I would succeed. I threw myself into my holistic health business and, within six months, I had a very long waiting list. I felt so blessed by it all. I never gave up on what was right by my conscience.

That was the beginning of a very special chapter in my business life, one which has grown and grown. I am now in my thirtieth year of practice, and run an expanded clinic.

Later that year, in 1994, I realised that I was pregnant again. Though it was unplanned, I was happy, as I love children. Little did I know how the outcome of that pregnancy would change my life forever.

And yet, my beautiful daughter Caoimhe has brought me such joy for the past twenty years.

Chapter 2
Best of Days, Worst of Days
10 July 1995

It was the summer of 1995, and my sixth baby was due on 30 July. My baby was to be delivered by elective caesarean section due to my previous obstetric history, so it was assumed by all concerned that I would be scheduled to give birth earlier in July. My delivery was to take place at Our Lady of Lourdes Hospital, Drogheda, as I had returned there for my confinement during this pregnancy from the Coombe Hospital, Dublin, where my previous two children had been delivered. As Dr Michael Neary's patient, my antenatal consultations took place at his private rooms in Fair Street, Drogheda. The ultrasound scans were frequently performed at the nearby Lourdes Hospital, as Neary did not have scanning facilities available at his private rooms. Frequent scanning as a means of foetal assessment was the new norm, unlike during my earlier pregnancies.

On 4 June 1995 I was admitted to the Lourdes Hospital, suffering from right-sided abdominal pain earlier that day. On examination, Neary stated that I had a rupture of my round ligament. The round ligament is the structure that holds the uterus and womb suspended inside the abdominal cavity. His statement was interesting in hindsight, as he came to the diagnosis using only abdominal palpitations as evidence, which is unusual.

Apart from clinically suspecting the condition, proper diagnosis is made and confirmed by an ultrasound scan and blood tests. No such testing was carried out following his diagnosis. I had numerous ultrasound scans performed at earlier stages of the pregnancy, but this latest revelation and recording would have warranted an up-to-date scan to confirm or refute his findings. This was not performed. Of course, the curiousness of his diagnosis did not occur to me at the time as I trusted Neary's competence and believed in him as my consultant. Any ideas about negligence or some other agenda did not enter my head then.

Interestingly, when I received my clinical notes years later, I learned that the verbal diagnosis he gave me was not *remotely* similar to what was written in my patient hospital records. Instead, the insertion in the chart reads: 'Right round ligament tenderness, uterus soft, CTG normal.'

CTG, or cardiotocography, is a test to check if the baby's heart is beating at a normal rate and variability. 'Tenderness' is certainly at variance with the diagnosis of 'rupture' that was given. Why would a doctor want to scare their patient so badly, unless for their own vile and twisted satisfaction?

Two weeks previous to this he had stated that I had placenta praevia, a condition in which the afterbirth is situated below or in front of the baby. In a normal delivery, the placenta or afterbirth is delivered after the birth of the baby – hence its name. In a vaginal delivery, however, where there is a placenta praevia condition, depending on its position, the placenta would be delivered before the baby once labour commences. This would warrant an immediate delivery by caesarean section to ensure the survival of the infant. This condition would be detected by ultrasound scan from very early on in the pregnancy. Since the placenta is the baby's 'lifeline', delivering it before the baby could lead to the death of the infant. The incidence of this condition is estimated to be four in one thousand. I was not unduly concerned, as I was due for a caesarean section anyway, and I had experienced a similar condition in my second pregnancy. But since the placenta is visible from early pregnancy I was curious as to why he had refrained from telling me this in the preceding months.

I was discharged home from hospital on 5 June 1995. Surely, if there was even the suspicion, much less a confirmation, of a ruptured round ligament I would have been detained in hospital for the remainder of my pregnancy, instead, I was discharged. Pregnant women are affected by vast hormonal changes which may distort their memories, and 'baby brain' can be common, even to the extent of not thinking coherently at times. Therefore, I did not question his decision to discharge me at the time. I was just glad to get home.

I was readmitted to hospital on 7 July, having had some bleeding at home, which I suspected was most likely due to the placenta praevia. I knew this could be an indication that the placenta was separating, and was a red flag in midwifery terms. On admission to the Lourdes Hospital, another ultrasound was performed after I voiced my concerns. On review Neary told me that he had seen placenta accreta on the latest ultrasound scan. He proceeded to tell me that he had scheduled the planned caesarean section for 10 July.

Placenta accreta occurs when the placenta attaches too deeply into the uterine wall but does not penetrate the uterine muscle.

The 'normal' placenta detaches from the uterine wall with relative ease during the third stage of the labour process. However, with placenta accreta it may require surgical removal to fully remove the placenta and stem the bleeding. In *some* cases it requires hysterectomy, *when it is impossible to detach the placenta because it has invaded the uterine wall too deeply*, or *where there is failure to stem the bleeding after all reasonable attempts to do so*. Bleeding can be excessive, as the placenta is a very vascular organ. The incidence of this condition is estimated to be 1.7 out of ten thousand pregnancies: it is a very rare occurrence.

Not having encountered or even heard of this condition during my midwifery training – probably due to its rarity – I enquired what it meant. Neary explained that the placenta was growing into the uterine wall, and that this 'sometimes' warranted hysterectomy. On hearing this I became very anxious and upset, as I did not want a hysterectomy. He sternly repeated, 'I said it *sometimes* means the outcome may be hysterectomy, I did not say that it will,' and he walked away with an angry look on his face. I knew I had crossed his boundaries.

My 'baby brain' again prevented me from thinking rationally or questioning him further at that time. But all these years on, I wonder why this had not been detected during earlier ultrasound scans, since this condition would have been evident from early pregnancy. God knows I had plenty of scans, so such abnormalities should have been apparent and reported on. At no time did any of the performing ultrasonographers ever mention a 'suspicion' of this condition being present. Of course, all the ultrasound reports were sent to Neary's private rooms, and that segment of my records has never been found. I learned years later that they mysteriously went missing when the inquiries began. During the antenatal consultations I had with Neary he never made reference to abnormal ultrasound findings, either of placenta praevia or placenta accreta. During each brief antenatal visit, his final analysis was: 'Everything is fine, see you in a few weeks.' I can only assume that either such diagnoses never appeared on those ultrasound reports, or Dr Neary did not read those reports, or that, for some reason, he chose to throw all the anomalies at me at an opportune time for him when I was most vulnerable and did not have time to research.

Having looked at the pathology report from the laboratory all these years on, it clearly states therein:

Sub-total post-partum hysterectomy: placental changes suggest intrauterine stress with some features consistent with placenta accreta but no adherent placental tissue seen. Cut surface, no abnormalities detected.

The report from the Review Group in April 1999 addressed their findings on Dr Neary's diagnosis of placenta accreta as follows:

The clinical diagnosis of a morbidly adherent placenta accreta was made in a number of patients at the time of operation. However, in retrospect, the clinical diagnosis of a morbidly adherent placenta was not confirmed histologically in *almost all of these patients* [my italics]. At interview, Dr Neary expressed several views as to why this had occurred, and he agreed that re-examination of the material by an independent specialist pathologist might clarify these differences. Dr Neary subsequently agreed to forego a review by an independent pathologist.

But even this not alter my later challenges for compensation. Whether or not there was an independent review carried out by a specialist pathologist, it was already too late for those of us who had suffered at the hands of his scalpel. What is the truth? We will probably never learn the real answers.

'Morbidly adherent placenta' indicates the surgical removal of the placenta, but not necessarily a hysterectomy as standard procedure. My pathology report, however, clearly states that it was not adherent. This would appear to suggest that while I may have had some degree of placenta accreta, there was no morbidly adherent tissue. Therefore, it seems it could have been removed without any surgical intervention, huge blood loss or hysterectomy. There certainly wasn't time allowed to see if any exceptional bleeding would stem itself, since he went on to delcare there to be massive blood loss before even delivering my baby. There was no real reason for the procedure, there was no exceptional bleeding.

I have met numerous women over the past nineteen years who have had placenta accreta in pregnancy, and who went on to have further babies. Fortunately for them, they were under the care of different consultants in different hospitals.

Had Neary already decided prenatally that I was to be his next victim?

10 July, a Black Day

The planned caesarean section was being performed under epidural anesthesia with the insertion and infusion of anaesthetic being commenced in theatre before Dr Neary arrived. This would have been the norm. There was nothing unusual noted or cited by the anaesthetist, nor did she make any reference to the multiple complications which Neary had relayed to me. Had any of this information been written in my chart she would have known, as she had access to my hospital clinical notes, which she shared with Neary. Being a woman and mother, one might imagine she would have made reference to the impending situation. I remember thinking it was odd at the time but accepting that the anaesthetist obviously had a very clear delineation of her job description. I remembered her from my student days, when I had known her as a very reserved individual who spoke little at the best of times.

Neary entered the theatre and immediately came to my side. He said: 'I will go in high with the incision to avoid holing your bladder. Your uterus is ruptured. The baby is lying outside the womb – he is lying on your bladder. You're in such a mess that I don't know what I'll find when I get in there.' Having made this declaration he walked away and began to scrub for surgery with his usual smirk, casually jesting with staff, as if all was well and this was just another routine procedure.

I was shocked by this news, and wondered when all this had been discovered. *Why was I not told about this before?* I thought. It now seemed to me that with each new conversation I was having with Neary, there were further adverse findings and more anticipated complications. I wondered if there were more revelations he was choosing not to tell me yet, and whether this was normal, or if it was his way of keeping me calm before theatre. As I was now anaesthetised, I could not move – it was a case of kicking someone when they were down. Nobody in the operating theatre spoke about what he had said, or addressed me to comment on it, reassuring me or otherwise. There I was, unable to move and with emotional paralysis setting in, and staff were going about their theatre duties as if all was well.

All the while, I assumed that Neary was trustworthy and competent. *It must be his findings that are causing him to make a high abdominal incision.* I trusted him. In a strange way I assumed – or hoped – that this was his way of protecting me from such serious news. But I felt truly terrified and alone, unsure of what I was facing. When all the standard theatre checks were complete, Neary asked the anaesthetist: 'Are we ready to go?'

Within seconds of his making the abdominal incision, Dr Neary shouted: 'Jesus, what have we got here? She'll bleed to death, there is blood everywhere – we are going to lose them both.' The assisting Senior House Officer neither replied nor altered his expression following Neary's declaration.

I started screaming, 'Don't let me die, don't let me die!' I was frantic with panic and fear. The sister midwife tried to insert earphones into my ears to prevent me from hearing the commotion, and tried to calm me down, but I pulled them off and continued to scream. The anaesthetist, who was positioned above my head, never spoke.

Neary turned towards me, saying, 'Kathleen, there's blood everywhere. I will have to do a hysterectomy in a hurry. I've got to cut right through your bladder, and I haven't reached the baby yet. It will be a miracle if he gets out alive. There's a big hole here. There's blood everywhere. We'll have to work fast to save your life.' At that point I must have wakened the dead in the cemetery across the road with my screaming.

Then he started shouting for clamps, and it felt like there was pandemonium everywhere. In hindsight I must have passed out at that stage, or was drifting in and out of a semi-conscious state as I felt my life was ebbing away rapidly.

I was crying profusely, and felt totally shocked. My entire life flashed before me, as I lay there anaesthetised from the waist down.

I was afraid to die.

I would never have a chance to say goodbye to my children or husband.

Who would rear and educate my children?

How would the family survive without me and my income?

What about my husband and parents? Who would tell them?

I had no reason to disbelieve Neary, so I thought that I must be about to die.

Then I remembered his previous statement, that the baby was lying on my bladder. I immediately thought that the profuse bleeding must be as a result of him cutting right through the baby, if he had indeed cut through my bladder, as he had said.

It all sounded so macabre that I felt physically sick. I felt like an astronaut being propelled into space, such was the speed of my changes in thought.

I was overcome by distress and panic.

My abiding memory of Neary at this juncture in the surgery was of the heavy beads of perspiration forming on his forehead and running down his face. He looked purple. Everybody else in theatre seemed composed, with an almost weird sense of normality, as if this were a routine occurrence. Nobody spoke during any of the proceedings.

He must be working really hard to save me, I thought. I lost track of time during the ensuing proceedings.

His facial expression remains as clearly etched in my mind's eye today as it was then. Reflecting on this, the profuse sweating could be interpreted as a sign of severe stress, even panic, but it also could have been a sign of excitement. *Yes!* he might have thought. *I've landed another coup!* Was he the self-appointed mouthpiece whenever he made such misguided decisions, so that all theatre staff knew better than to speak out?

Nineteen years on, my impression of him is even more clear: he was like a starving dog drooling over a juicy T-bone steak: *I* was his juicy T-bone steak, on that day.

Was he having a panic attack, or simply acting like a vulture in full flight? How could any doctor think it was necessary to perform a hysterectomy before they had reached the uterus?

Neary finally lifted up my baby, saying, 'You've got another little girl; she must be a survivor because it's a miracle she's still alive. I just hope she will be okay because you should both be dead.'

I do not even remember being handed my baby, how long I held her or who took her from me, such was my distress. My mind felt like I was in a speeding rally car. I have no recollection of being sutured, what he said or what his appearance or demeanour was like after that, until I was being wheeled out of theatre.

Neary was at the head of the trolley as they were transferring me to the recovery room next door. As the theatre doors opened, Peter was standing there. Knowing him from the deliveries of our previous children in Drogheda, Neary extended his hand, saying: 'Congratulations Peter, you've got a baby daughter. We have christened her "Miracle" because they should both be dead, but for now they are both alive. Kathleen nearly bled to death in there. There was blood everywhere. I had a tough job saving her life. She gave us a hell of a fright. Neither of them are out of the woods yet. For now they are both alive, but they should both be dead.'

Peter thanked him profusely, and later went into downtown Drogheda to buy him a piece of Waterford glass as a token of gratitude for saving our lives.

Of course, our daughter was not christened in theatre, nor was she ever called 'Miracle'.

If my daughter was indeed so close to death, then:

1. She should not have reached her Apgar score of seven at one minute. An Apgar score is a method of evaluating the newborn infant using five simple criteria: appearance, pulse, grimace, activity, respiration. It is reassessed at five minutes after birth. A score of seven at one minute is regarded as satisfactory, with a score of ten at five minutes regarded as normal. My daughter's score was seven at one minute and ten at five minutes, which was not indicative of the near-death infant she was deemed to have been by Dr Neary. Her paediatric notes make no reference to a 'near-death infant', not even an infant in distress.

2. If she was, as he had stated, lying on my bladder, how did he avoid making an incision right through her little body when he made his rash cut straight through my bladder?

3. Surely if all these complications had been noted since 4 June I should have been bleeding and in pain, with my vital signs failing in the interim: they were not. I should have been closely monitored in hospital I should think. Equally, my baby should have been exhibiting signs of foetal distress: she was not. One does not walk around comfortably, if at all, with a ruptured uterus, especially for six weeks. Yet I was performing normal daily activities at home with my family and at work during this time.

4. Why did my vital signs (blood pressure and pulse) remain completely stable if I was bleeding so profusely? These vital signs – pulse and blood pressure – would normally drop drastically and continually during haemorrhage unless corrective measures were instituted. No such measures were applied, presumably as they were not required. Given that I normally have a low blood pressure even in a non-pregnant state, I would have passed out quickly.

5. Why was a blood transfusion not deemed necessary, especially since I had already been told that I was anaemic? Blood had been cross-matched, and was available in theatre on that day. The cross-matching of blood before surgery is a routine measure to ensure the correct blood group is available. But a blood transfusion was neither mentioned nor considered. It was not needed, because I was not bleeding profusely. My total blood loss recorded in my notes was 1,000 millilitres, which is normal blood loss following a caesarean section.

6. Why was my haemoglobin (iron level) recorded as similar pre/post-operatively at 10.6 g/dl?

7. If I was bleeding so profusely on incision and it was
    impossible to perform the hysterectomy until after the
    baby's delivery, given the time factor involved, the
    blood loss would potentially have to be several pints,
    as the contracted uterus would pump out blood rap-
    idly. Instead, it was normal.

When I was a pupil midwife at the Lourdes Hospital, all pregnant women were expected to sign a consent form on admission, irrespective of their stage in pregnancy or labour: this was
the rule. The explanation that we as students were given was;
should a pregnant woman require anaesthetic at any stage during her stay in hospital for any procedure, including emergency
caesarean section, manual removal of placenta or anything else,
she could legally claim later that she was not of sound mind at
the time if the form signed in an emergency situation. I too
signed such a consent form on 9 July.

In my case, however, on receipt of my clinical notes years
later, I noticed 'T.A.H.' (total abdominal hysterectomy) had
been added to my signature, or more accurately, the addition
had been forged. I know for certain that this was not written
on the form when I signed.

As I previously stated, hysterectomy as a possible consequence of placenta accreta had been mentioned to me, but, as I
understood it, this was not the expressed or intended outcome.
So why would it have been written before surgery? I am certain
it was not written on the form at the time of my signing. When
was 'T.A.H.' added, by whom and on whose instructions? Was
this part of the 'chart altering' that Judge Maureen Harding
Clark would refer to years later in her summation?

Chapter 3
When Am I Going to Die?

Having spent time in the recovery room, as was routine procedure following surgery, I was wheeled back to the ward, still reeling with shock. The recovery room is next to theatre, and is where all patients are closely monitored in the immediate aftermath of all surgeries. Peter had gone downtown to get the thank-you gift for Dr Neary. When he returned I did not even want to speak to him. *Even he walked out on me in my dying moments*, I thought. Peter was full of gratitude for our survival, and tried to reassure me, reiterating how great Dr Neary was. But I felt that Peter did not fully comprehend that I could soon die. *He obviously did not fully hear what Neary had said*, was my immediate thought. Bonding with my beautiful daughter – what good was that? I was not going to be here for much longer and my death was imminent, according to Dr Neary. My daughter was in the special care unit anyway, so it was best I did not see her as I could not bear to part with her again. Babies were placed in the special care baby unit as a routine procedure within the hospital for observation, following any caesarean-section delivery, amongst other reasons.

As I peered at the catheter drainage bag I noticed it was full of bright red blood, and seemed to be filling up fast. *So he was right*, I thought. *There was blood everywhere*. It looked as if my life was ebbing away through this catheter hanging by the side of the bed, and nobody was taking any notice. I was bleeding to death, and no one cared.

Physical pain is one thing, but emotional anguish is indescribable: waiting to die, afraid to go asleep lest I never wake up again, or, worse, wake up in a 'foreign country' that I was not yet ready for and did not want to go to yet. I don't even remember the physical pain after the operation as it was probably well controlled. But physical pain was also really secondary to my emotional state at that moment, and that pain was raging. Peter showered me with gifts but I was not remotely interested in opening them – I didn't think I'd get the chance to use them. The solitude was fearful.

Nobody had mentioned death. *How can they be so detached, so cold?* I wondered. *Surely this could not be routine?* I thought. *Surely I should have a nurse with me at all times?* I know that I would have always stayed with a dying patient, throughout my nursing career. Of course, when I had access to my hospital notes years later, I realised that none of the drama in the theatre had been included in the chart entry by Neary following surgery. Ward staff could not have known what I was fearing. Instead his insertion read:

Repeat classical caesarean section, sub-total hysterectomy, repair of bladder. Placenta praevia, placenta accreta whole right side of uterus, incomplete rupture two-inch hole in bladder. Bladder forming lower segment of uterus. I do not know when bladder was holed but it was quite impossible to avoid putting hole in bladder.

The addition of the 'hole in my bladder' seems contradictory in itself: either he did not know when it was holed or he made the hole himself, as he had told me.

So one can only deduce that either the ward staff did not know about the traumatic incident first-hand, or they were so accustomed to hearing of such inflated theatrics that it was an accepted norm they chose to ignore, or at least not speak out about. Perhaps there may even have been a decision at ward level not to discuss such events with the patient, in the hope that it had 'gone right over their head' and they did not understand what he had said. Perhaps they had forgotten that I too was a qualified midwife.

Scary thoughts kept racing round and round in my head. Neary was off-duty for the next few days so I felt there was no one with any authority to discuss what was happening, or from whom I could seek answers.

Within a few days I began having nightmares about dying and about the hysterectomy, dreaming that my baby had been butchered to death. In my dream I was looking down at my own dead body and my little daughter's butchered, dismembered, lifeless frame. One nightmare terrified me for days: I dreamt that I was inside a coffin, clawing so hard at the sides to get out that I scratched away the timber interior. I would wake up screaming several times each night.

These dreams became deeply disturbing for me, and I asked nursing staff if I could speak with a counsellor. I wasn't sure if I was still dying or simply going mad. I repeated this request to numerous staff nurses, but despite them giving me an affirmative each time, it seemed to fall on deaf ears. Despite their assurances, my fears were reinforced by my conviction that nobody was brave enough to tell me to my face that I was going to die. I thought perhaps that they were taking palliative measures.

Several days later the hospital matron came to see me, referred to by the accompanying ward sister as the 'counsellor'. She had been matron at the hospital back in 1978, when I was a pupil midwife. She was not a counsellor, to my knowledge. She may have been a wonderful midwife and a great matron, but I wondered whether a woman who had never given birth could really understand my situation. Such was my train of thought as she sat down to 'counsel' me. My experience with her is not meant as a slight upon her character in either a professional or personal capacity.

She was a very nice, proper and serious lady. She sat across the room, looking very composed. She did not speak much about what had happened in theatre. Apart from some initial small talk, she did not ask how I was feeling, nor did she once mention death. She had little to say about the ordeal. I would have expected all of these topics to be discussed by a counsellor. I only remember brief snippets of our conversation, as I 'tuned out' in my fury at her being sent to see me as the counsellor. I am not sure if she really knew why she was counselling me, or whether she was instead sidestepping the issue. Her advice was theoretically wonderful but not practical from what I had been through or was now experiencing. She said: 'You have your complete family now. Put the past behind you, go home and get on with your life.'

If only life could fit snugly into such compartments for all of us.

But as I know now, as a past matron, perhaps this lady had expressed concern some years before over the number of hysterectomies being performed by Neary. Back then her concern might have fallen on deaf ears. Perhaps in her own quiet way, she was now empathasising with my situation, whether or not she was fully aware of what he had said in theatre. After all, she may perhaps once again have been witnessing a hysterectomy being unnecessarily performed and notched up within the hospital records. I feel sure that, if she understood any of what was happening, she did not like the legacy she was witnessing at a hospital she had devoted her life to. If she indeed suspected what was going on, her professionalism would not allow her, to make such an admission. As she left the room I cried tears of anger and hurt. I had made the request for counselling to help the healing process, if I was indeed going to live. I remember shouting, 'Jesus, will somebody please listen to me?' Being in a single room, of course, nobody could hear me scream.

In my experience of hospital-patient management, there is great emphasis on keeping the patient physically pain-free, but emotional healing does not appear to come into the remit within the medical model. It is almost as though 'brain pain' is unrecognised in allopathic medicine – at least that is exactly how it was in my experience. I wonder if much has really changed in that area. I hear similar stories related to me by clients daily in my own practice, about their various emotional concerns not being addressed in allopathic medicine. But 'brain pain' is the most damaging, powerful and dangerous pain of all.

However, I do know of many caring doctors who have trained in psychotherapy, cognitive behavioural therapy, mindfulness and other methods of emotional healing, which they incorporate into their practice.

On the day of my discharge, Dr Neary was off duty. He was replaced by another consultant obstetrician, who was covering Neary's schedule. He arrived with his entourage of registrars and junior doctors to certify my discharge. As was his usual demeanour, he was flamboyant and blasé, jesting with the junior doctors. The staff midwife advised him of my request for counselling and informed him that the matron had spoken with me. He looked at me with a dismissive, curious smirk, as if I was from another planet.

As he turned to leave the room, he allowed his accompanying doctors to exit before him. Then he turned back to me, halfway out the door, and said: 'I don't know what you are worrying about, Kathleen – at least you will never be back here having more babies.'

He closed the door, and his laughter rang loudly in my ears as he proceeded down the corridor. That statement cut through me as deeply as Neary's scalpel. I felt like hurling something at the door in frustration. Instead, I lay crying into my pillow.

I was deeply aggrieved by his callous sarcasm, and later complained to numerous staff nurses. My complaints seemingly fell on deaf ears, and were, of course, never mentioned again. I feel that such was the deference given to doctors at that time, that nurses felt unable or unwilling to comment. How could anybody, much less a doctor, be so insensitive to a patient, and particularly after what I had experienced? I had come through a near-death experience, as Neary had said. I had undergone what is, to me, the most invasive female surgery imaginable, and the best he could offer was to jest at my misfortune. His insensitivity did not, however, surprise me: I had experienced his attitude during my second pregnancy.

Dr Neary phoned me at home a few days later, asking why I had requested counselling. I thought it was unusual to receive such a call, but at the time I also felt that he must be a caring doctor to follow up on discharged patients by telephoning them at home. I explained that I feared going into a postnatal depression following the trauma I had experienced, and the resonance and reality of this – very much ongoing – trauma. After all, I had more than a little knowledge and experience in this area, having been a midwife and antenatal tutor for many years. I had suffered from postnatal depression following the birth of my second baby so, in an effort to avoid a repeat of this situation, I was trying to be prophylactic in my early request for help. I explained to him how I needed to make a full recovery as quickly as possible, as I now had six children and needed to get back to work quickly for financial and familial reasons. I simply wanted to be well, and could not afford to give a minute to illness.

He dismissed my fears, and said that he would see me in his rooms in Fair Street in six weeks.

Neary's call did little to allay my ongoing sense of terror.

Chapter 4
My Obstetric History

I had worked with Dr Neary both during my general nurse training as a student nurse and, later, as a pupil midwife. He was the busiest of all the consultants working in the International Medical Missionary Training Hospital, Drogheda, also known as the Lourdes Hospital. Perhaps he took on an extra caseload, as he was also the youngest of the three consultants there at that time, having being appointed a consultant at the age of thirty-one. Either he was very brilliant, or he had cleverly wormed his way into the position, or, perhaps it had been a little of both. He often stayed overnight in the hospital if a number of his patients were actively in labour, which added to his image was a wonderfully caring doctor. He was always smartly dressed, in grey trousers and a navy blazer: it was his uniform. In my extreme naivety, I assumed that he must be the best obstetrician and gynaecologist in the hospital. Discussions about consultants or their activities never featured in our training, nor did we feel entitled to be privy to such information. Instead, we were advised to be attentive, and never to question suggested outcomes, as the consultant always knew best.

From working with him, I knew he had a quirky sense of humour. In my early training days, nobody was allowed to call another staff or student member by their Christian name – you were referred to as 'Nurse' and your surname. But as very new students in the general hospital, he insisted on knowing our Christian names and addressing us by them. This terrified us, as we feared being strongly reprimanded or even expelled if this happened within earshot of anyone else, especially the Medical Missionary Sisters. He would come to the student cafeteria, often when we were on night duty, and insist on joining in on student conversations. In those days, many students used to knit during their break time. He would take the knitting from the student and became an authority on whatever piece they were making, showing them different stitches and so on. He told us about growing up in Ballina in County Mayo, and how he was reared by his grandmother, whom he described as the local herbalist, who made her own herbal potions. We were never made aware of his family situation, nor did we ask why he was reared by his grandmother. So full of fear were we of the system that prevailed that we listened to what we were told, and did not ask questions. Neary told us how he had worked in London, Portsmouth and Manchester before taking up his position in Drogheda. He also talked about his wife Gabriel, and their three children. He could be personable and friendly.

There were many strange incidents that occurred when I was working with him. He could be incredibly nice to patients, and then suddenly switch to being very rude. He was especially heavy-handed in theatre, and appeared to poke around the abdomen of the mother when performing a caesarean section, unlike the other two obstetricians. His explanation was that he was 'having a general root around to check everything'. It is no small wonder that his patients complained of greater pain in the post-operative period than mothers who had their surgery performed by other obstetricians. But as a student – and I was just that, 'a student' – I thought that because he was the consultant, he must be right. Nobody seemed to publicly question anything, especially the regular theatre staff. If they did question anything, it was never discussed with us students.

When I realised that I was pregnant with my first daughter, in 1982, I had automatically booked Dr Neary for my antenatal and perinatal care in a private-patient capacity, as I had VHI insurance. The pregnancy was largely uneventful, and the delivery was assisted by use of a forceps. The post-partum period was uneventful.

In my second pregnancy I also booked Dr Neary for my care. At that time, in 1984, regular performance of ultrasound scans during pregnancy was not the norm, unless something untoward was suspected. This pregnancy was uneventful until ten days before my estimated date of delivery. Peter, Arlene and I were on holidays in Bundoran, County Donegal. I realised that I had stopped 'feeling life' inside of me: that is, I could not feel the baby move. I became alarmed, and felt like something was wrong. It was a mother's intuition, I suppose. We decided to cut our holiday short and come home. On our journey back to Monaghan I remained conscious of the absence of my baby's kicks. I even stayed up all night to check. I went to see my GP the next morning, using his stethoscope, he had concluded that everything was fine, and said that he could find the baby's heartbeat. While he was very reassuring, he was acutely aware of how concerned I was. To reassure me further, he suggested that I go to the hospital and request to have an ultrasound scan to give me peace of mind. I decided to follow this advice, and immediately went to the Lourdes Maternity Hospital for a check-up. I could not get the line that I had been taught as a pupil midwife out of my head: pregnancy is abnormal until mother and baby are safely delivered. This line was frequently trotted out by one of my tutor midwives during my training days, the memory of which I was, and am, acutely aware of.

I learned that Dr Neary was on holiday that week when I got to the hospital, but I was seen by another obstetrician, who was covering his duty for the weekend.

The old Lourdes Maternity Hospital, while on the same grounds as the General Hospital, was situated on the opposite side of the Medical Missionaries convent. Being quite an old building, it did not have a lift, but had a flight of stairs and a small landing, then a second flight of stairs, along which all admissions ascended. As I approached the landing, a sister midwife whom I knew was standing at the top of the stairs with a man. She greeted me from the top landing and explained to the doctor that I had been a former midwifery student there. He greeted me with profound rudeness. 'Ah, so you are the fussy midwife sent in from Ballybay,' he said.

Following an examination, he insisted that there was nothing amiss and that I was imagining things. I should go home, he said, as there were no beds available. Normally timid, I stuck my heels in and told him, 'I am going nowhere.' He was obviously incensed, but I remained strong in my conviction in my maternal instinct. I knew that there was something amiss. I knew that I needed to stay assertive for my unborn baby. I requested an ultrasound scan, but he dismissed me. He called it an 'unnecessary intervention', and refused to consent. Even though I protested, and said that I was prepared to pay for the ultrasound scan as a private patient, he continued to refuse, and repeated his advice that I should go home. I insisted that I was prepared to sit and wait if necessary, but that I wanted to stay within the precincts of the hospital. He was disgusted. I could overhear him complaining to staff about 'that bloody, fussy midwife'. To this day, I do not know where my inner strength came from, but it must have been God-sent. Marianne Williamson says: 'Our deepest fear is not that we are inadequate; our deepest fear is that we are powerful beyond measure. It is our light, not our darkness, that most frightens us.'

*

It was one of those beautiful sunny summer days, during the heatwave of 1984. The staff nurse told me to sit out on the veranda as there were no available beds. There were also other mothers-to-be there in varying stages of their pregnancies, just out enjoying the pleasant weather.

I was handed a 'kick chart' to record foetal movement, but this was why I was there in the first place: I could not feel life within me. I protested to the nurse, but it went unheeded. What was the point in me holding onto a kick chart if I was not feeling any movement? I wondered.

After about an hour on the veranda, I was told by a midwife that they had located a bed for me downstairs in St Brigid's Ward, to which I was duly taken. This ward was for women experiencing obstetric difficulties in the antenatal period. Some ladies there had spent most of their pregnancy in hospital for various obstetric conditions, especially older first-time mothers. This was the one ward in the hospital I had disliked during my training days. It was old, dull and dark, and almost always had a fusty smell.

In 1984 few were privileged with mobile phones, so I went to the public coin box and called Peter. I remember saying: 'Maybe I should have gone home. I don't know what I am doing here, but I don't feel right.' Peter was busy baling hay, and said he may not get to the hospital that night as they would be working late. I returned to my bed and, within a few minutes, during a conversation with one of the long-term patients, I thought that my 'waters' must have broken – I felt saturated. But when I investigated further, I realised that I was bleeding profusely, and the bed was covered in blood. I had suffered a massive haemorrhage. I screamed so loudly that they heard me upstairs in the labour ward, and staff came running to investigate. Bells rang everywhere, and I was put in theatre for an emergency caesarean section within fifteen minutes. I was put in the emergency lift to descend to the ground floor, where the theatre was situated. In this frightening lift, the patient's torso was pushed under a lower part of the antiquated chamber. Its descent of one flight seemed to take forever: it was like being in a tomb. I remember the elderly priest running along the corridor beside me, praying, as staff ran down the corridor towards the theatre, pushing me on the trolley. The priest was told he had no time to give me the last rites, such was the level of the perceived emergency.

As we entered the theatre, the doctor said, 'I'm sure you are glad you stayed.' This statement came from a man who, a couple of hours earlier, was determined to send me home. I replied:

'For all our sakes, I am sure you are glad I stayed – you had better not let me die.' This was how I felt, irrespective of how fearful I was at that time.

As it was an emergency caesarean section, there was no time to contact anybody, so I was terrified and on my own undergoing an emergency surgery with general anaesthetic. All I had known about this doctor was that a mother from a neighbouring parish had died during a caesarean section that he had performed that same year. My immediate thoughts as I was 'run' into theatre that evening were not positive. I remember precious little after this, as I was immediately put under general anaesthetic in preparation for surgery.

The message herein is: always listen to your maternal instinct. Irrespective of what you are being told by others, you know your body better than anyone.

★

After the caesarean section was performed and I exited the recovery room, I was taken back to the postnatal ward, where I was told that the reason for the haemorrhage was a condition called placenta praevia. Had my earlier pleas for an ultrasound scan been heard, this frightening emergency could have been averted, and I could have had a routine, albeit emergency, caesarean section performed hours earlier. I had apparently haemorrhaged so profusely in theatre that I had to have four units of blood transfused. As I live thirty-five miles from the hospital, and it was in the days before the motorway to Monaghan existed, I feel sure that I would have died, such was the extent of the haemorrhaging.

My baby had breathed some of the blood into her lungs, and was very ill. She spent several days in the special care baby unit. When I regained consciousness following my surgery, I kept asking to see my baby. I was repeatedly told they would bring her in 'shortly'. I was given scant information as to the seriousness of her condition, but I later learned from the paediatrician that, at many intervals, they were concerned for her survival. It was almost twenty hours before I got to see or hold Karen, my beautiful daughter. Early bonding was broken with her because of a doctor ignoring his patient.

Interestingly, when Dr Neary returned from his weekend off, his emphasis was not on the fact that he had failed to diagnose placenta praevia during my antenatal care. Instead, he said that I had given the theatre staff 'one hell of a fright', as I had experienced cardiac arrest during surgery and had had to be resuscitated.

This frightened and baffled me, as neither Dr Lynch nor any nursing staff had made any reference in the post-operative period to cardiac arrest. The accompanying nurse on his consultant rounds made no comment on this, either then or later.

Assuming he was referring to antepartum haemorrhage, I replied: 'If Dr Lynch had listened to me, this could have been averted.' But he re-emphasised his earlier statement that I had suffered from cardiac arrest, and had had to be resuscitated. In some strange way at the time, I managed to rationalise this happening with the sudden extreme blood loss I had suffered.

I subsequently found there to be no record of his startling proclamations in my clinical notes. I can only deduce that this was another figment of his imagination: another desire to dramatise. It never happened, of course. It was all a sham, an egotistical solo run which, for whatever personal, twisted reason, he enjoyed.

When I asked him if I could take tests to ascertain whether I had had an allergic reaction to any component of the anaesthetic, he replied: 'There are no such tests. There is no such thing as an allergy here.' I did not question his authority, nor did I pursue it further, though I felt bothered by this response.

In hindsight, I wonder whether Dr Neary had been on duty that fateful night in 1984 when I had experienced such a massive haemorrhage, would I have then ended up with a hysterectomy? Each time I ponder this, I imagine the loss of all my future beautiful children, who I would have missed out on forever.

This was followed, within a few weeks, by a breast abscess, which warranted my being hospitalised. I then went into a severe postnatal depression lasting for several months. Of course, what I did not realise at the time was that the major contributing factor to all of this was the shock I had endured. Fortunately, I was able to be treated at home and on an outpatient basis for the postnatal depression. It was a horribly frightening period in my life.

My third pregnancy was overdue by ten days. Labour had to be induced and surgically commenced. Following the induction, and even after privately ingesting a horrible bottle of castor oil, I did not satisfactorily progress to labour. Once again, this meant that I had to have an emergency caesarean section under general anaesthetic, performed by Neary.

Afterwards, he repeated: 'You had a close brush with death in there last night. You "arrested" again. I had to work fast to save your life.' When I further questioned him to ascertain the possible cause of the cardiac arrest, he went on to suggest that

I must have some sort of phobia about anaesthetics.

Again, I asked if there was a test for a possible allergy to a component of the anaesthetic. Since my previous delivery in 1984, I had watched an RTÉ documentary on severe reactions to anaesthetics, which I related to him. His reply was: 'Nonsense, get treated for the phobia.' However, no further treatment was suggested or recommended.

In my entire career, I have never heard of a phobia causing cardiac arrest. I have researched this extensively, and cannot find any substantive evidence to support his claim.

This second supposed cardiac arrest was also not recorded in my notes.

In my fourth pregnancy, I decided to go to the Coombe Maternity Hospital, in Dublin, for delivery. I knew I would have to be delivered by caesarean section because of my obstetric history. But as I still thought that there was an anaesthetic problem, with increased risk of repeat cardiac arrest, I assumed an epidural anaesthetic might be a safer option. At this time, epidural anaesthesia was not an option at the Lourdes Hospital, but was available at the Coombe Hospital.

This delivery was an uneventful caesarean section, as was the delivery of my fifth baby, at the same hospital and by the same consultant. My experience there was very different: so caring and compassionate. There was no drama, there were no theatrics. I remember, on my first visit, how the consultant listened intently as I recounted my story and voiced my serious concerns. She sat and listened, making no comment. I feel sure she must have had grave suspicions either about the veracity of the story I was relaying – or because she had heard similar tales before. Otherwise I feel sure she would have requested my hospital records from Drogheda. To my knowledge, this did not happen. To reassure me, she took me to visit a lady who had had seven babies, all delivered by caesarean section using epidural anaesthesia.

Both of the pregnancies I went to the Coombe for had uneventful postnatal periods, except for experiencing residual leg weakness after the fifth delivery. I was admitted to the Lourdes Hospital for investigations as I was falling frequently. Ironically, one evening as Peter was leaving the hospital he met Neary on the corridor. Neary enquired what he was doing at the hospital, so Peter explained. Neary's reply was: 'Ah sure, there are over one hundred side effects to epidural anaesthetics. That is why I never touch them.' Strange, then, that he later succumbed to working with epidural anaesthesia as the preferred anaesthetic procedure for caesarean sections.

When I found out that I was pregnant with my sixth child, I learned that epidural anaesthesia had become an option at the Lourdes Hospital. I returned to Dr Neary for my care, as Drogheda was much nearer to home, and would make my antenatal care easier.

What a mistake.

Chapter 5
I Went in to Have My Baby,
I Came out an Emotional Cripple

After the events of 10 July 1995, I remained emotionally disturbed and distressed, and experienced a number of health concerns. I was extremely tired – the sort of tiredness that any amount of sleep never resolved. I was initially told that it was probably due to anaemia, but as my iron level improved, my mood and extreme tiredness did not. The level of deep fatigue was immeasurable. I had horrendous nightmares, and cried a lot. My mood was like a kite in a hurricane. I experienced bowel and bladder problems, and was never well, moving from one symptom to the next. I felt detached from my husband, from my family and children. I felt detached from life itself, and even from myself. I felt split right down the middle. I had entered the Lourdes Hospital to give birth, but had come out an emotional cripple, without a glimmer of hope in sight for the future.

I went back to Dr Neary's rooms in Fair Street, Drogheda, for my six-week postnatal check-up. When Mrs Neary answered the door, she said, 'You are two weeks early.' That is an indicator of how distressed and confused I was. I was in a state of panic, which I did not recognise at the time.

I burst into tears. She asked me to take a seat in the waiting room, while she checked if Dr Neary could see me. There was one waiting room in this building where prenatal women, post-natal women and women with gynaecological problems all sat together, waiting for their appointment.

I entered and then exited the waiting room within the same minute. I said to Mrs Neary, 'Please don't put me in there with pregnant women.' She did not question why, but offered me a seat in the hallway. I remember shaking like a leaf. What was I so terrified of? I have no idea. I sat there, face turned towards the wall, afraid beyond belief, with tears streaming down my face.

After what seemed like hours but was probably scarcely thirty minutes, I was ushered into Dr Neary's consulting room. He reiterated the surgical complexities he had encountered on performing the caesarean section on 10 July. He repeated how hard he had worked to save my life, and thanked me for the gift that Peter had given him, saying how much he appreciated it.

He repeatedly stressed how lucky the baby and I were to be alive, after what he had encountered.

He told me that he had mistakenly cut through my bladder, but when he realised he had done this, he made an even *bigger* hole, as it was 'easier to stitch a big hole than a small one'. He casually told me: 'You might have some bladder problems such as incontinence and frequency of urination, but that is a small price to pay for having saved your life.'

He instructed me to immediately commence hormone-replacement therapy (HRT), and proceeded to write me a prescription for a drug called Premarin. He maintained that my distress was hormonal.

As I mentioned earlier, his chart insertion on 'holing my bladder' does not match with what he relayed to me. It would therefore appear to me that he made a false insertion in my notes post-surgery. It never dawned on me then that he was not 'supposed' to have removed my ovaries, and I should not have needed hormone-replacement therapy at all, especially so soon after a hysterectomy.

I stood up to leave, and proceeded to the door. As I placed my hand on the doorknob, he was still sitting at his desk. He turned to me and made an amazing statement, with his classic, jocular laugh: 'Kathleen, I have done you a big favour, you know. Now you can have sex without any fear of getting pregnant, and no more babies.'

He was still chuckling as I exited the room.

★

The drive home that day was dangerous. I passed sections of road without recollection, not knowing whether I was coming or going, not knowing what was going on, or going wrong, in my head. *Why would he make such a statement as I was leaving*, I thought. *Was he trying to be funny or to defuse the situation?*

Within a few days of starting the hormone replacement therapy, I felt much worse. I had sweats and hot flushes, was increasingly irritable, had headaches, and even had bleeding from my bowel movements. Additionally, I was not comfortable about taking the drug I had been prescribed, Premarin, as I was aware that it was made from the urine of pregnant mares. Ingesting this was nauseating at best, but I would have borne it if it had helped. Instead it made me feel worse.

I returned to Neary within the week. He discontinued the

hormone-replacement therapy (the horse urine) and put me on Prozac instead, now asserting that I was depressed. This new drug had absolutely no positive effect on how I was feeling. It just put a new label on an already hopeless situation.

As September rolled on, I remained exhausted and very unwell. But I knew that I had to return to work as I was now my family's main earner. I had just got the children back to school, and there were all the additional school bills that needed to be met. Money was scarce since I was not working, which increased my worries. Truth be told, I often worried where the next day's meals would come from. Every day was a struggle, but I returned to work at the end of September because I had to. I was (and am) self-employed, running a holistic health clinic, so I did not qualify for any paid sick leave, disability allowance or social-welfare payments.

I would often have to be in bed by 7 PM to be relatively functional by the next day, such were my levels of exhaustion. In hindsight, I now recognise that this was also a primary means of isolation. Cutting myself off from family and friends was part of a deeper condition. But I limped on and on through the ensuing months, feeling more and more depleted. There were times when I felt like I must be dying.

Christmas came, and I developed pleurisy, a debilitating lung condition. I was very ill. This left me spending most of the Christmas holidays in bed, and feeling extremely unwell.

January and February were dreadful months for me, healthwise. I was mentally exhausted, experiencing severe and repeated panic attacks, and feeling weepy, anxious and alone. I was also physically exhausted, and seemed to perpetually be either coming out of some illness or going into one. Nobody could give me any proper answers as to what was going on in my life.

★

On 16 March 1996 we had planned to visit my parents in Kerry for the weekend of St Patrick's Day. All our things were packed and everybody was in the car, including our six children.

Apparently, I left the car and returned to the house. I have no recollection of this. After ten minutes, Peter said that he came to investigate where I had gone, and found me banging my head off the bedroom wall, repeatedly saying: 'I can't cope, I can't go on.' He later told me that I was screaming so loudly that he feared I had been attacked. He repeatedly attempted to get me into the car, mistakenly thinking that I would 'snap out of it' when I got to Kerry. When his efforts failed, he put me to bed, annoyingly disbelieving how ill I was. He felt that I was disappointing the children, my parents and everyone around me. But I felt incapable of doing anything. I had imploded.

Peter could not bear to see me sick. His ability to cope with illness is fragile; it makes him very fearful. He is the youngest of seven children, one child having died aged three. His mother suffered from ill health for most of her life, and so for most of his childhood. She spent long periods in hospital. Being the youngest in his family, he opted to take over her role, both in the house and on the farm. It led to his early departure from school, either as an opportune excuse, or out of a perceived necessity.

In an unconscious way, he connected my being unwell with

his childhood experience, and could not revisit that painful era of his life. He was terrified. It was as if he was again faced with having to rear six children single-handedly, just like during his childhood. In essence, he could not cope either.

My abiding memory of that March day was how I wished that I could die. I locked the bedroom door in an attempt to shut out the world. I lay awake all night, crying and confused, with all sorts of frightening thoughts entering my head. Tears are amazing, one of God's wonderful gifts. As I lay there in distress, it was as if the dam had burst. The waterfalls of tears gave me a release, albeit a temporary one, which nothing else could accomplish. As they flowed out, they released some of the past months of hurt and inexplicable distress, cleansing me for a short while in the process. Although there was a large residue of hurt remaining to be dealt with, crying temporarily made it seeming easier to tackle.

The next day was an attempt to keep life 'normal'. Peter took the kids to the local St Patrick's Day parade, as they were obviously disappointed at not having gone to Kerry. I am sure they were also frightened, not understanding what was going on with their mother. I drank two large whiskeys to try to get some sleep, but this did not help. Again I was filled with anguish, tears tumbling down my cheeks until my skin felt like it was on fire. I could not eat; it was as if food was poisoning and suffocating me. Another night of ghastly anxiety followed, with much more crying and further sleeplessness. I remained on my own by choice. I thought that morning would never come. I was truly going through the dark night of the soul. The following day I called my GP, but I could not face telling Peter, lest he misunderstand.

I was scared of everything and everybody. My thinking had become warped.

I felt suicidal. I did not want to die, but I could not cope with living. Life felt completely over for me. I felt dead inside. I knew that I could not go on like this.

My GP came on a house visit and, as usual, behaved kindly, gently and compassionately. Having spent a long time listening to me, he calmly explained that I needed to be hospitalised for my own safety. He arranged an emergency appointment with the local psychiatric hospital, which I attended the following day. Peter was very startled and frightened by this, and cried profusely, questioning whether it was really necessary.

I attended the appointment as arranged. The psychiatrist agreed that I needed immediate hospitalisation, until my mental state had stabilised. I had worked at that particular psychiatric hospital in the past, and was not anxious to be admitted there as an inpatient. This seems ridiculous, in hindsight, but I worried that, because Ireland feels like such a small place, people love to gossip about others' woes.

Having spoken to the psychiatrist in the local hospital, and accepting that I needed immediate hospitalisation, my GP set about organising my admission to St Patrick's Psychiatric Hospital in Dublin, as soon as a bed could be arranged. In a strange way I felt relieved, as I needed to get well quickly and return to work. I desperately wanted a 'quick fix' – a magic wand.

Peter was initially not pleased with the doctor's recommendations, and did not accept them. He genuinely did not appreciate how ill I was – or he was too frightened to believe my state, as he felt that I was mirroring his childhood experiences. In a practical sense, he now had six young children to care for, and he felt incapable of doing this, and daunted by doing it alone.

His parents were both deceased, and mine lived in Kerry, so there was no readily available family help. It was a very tough period for all concerned.

Chapter 6
Psychiatry or Institutionalisation?

Later in that cold March week of 1996, I was given a date for my admission to St Patrick's Hospital. I had no idea where in Dublin I was going, nor did I care much, initially. I had heard of this hospital, but had not had any occasion to visit it or learn where it was located.

Leaving home that day was very matter-of-fact. I do not recall much conversation on that journey with Peter: it was mostly silence interspersed with tears from both of us.

As we turned in to the hospital driveway, the building seemed modern and bright, but this was only the front of house. We parked close to the reception area and entered those revolving doors. It was well-decorated with nice flowers and smelled of fresh paint, but that was where the brightness ended for me. The patient area was a stark reminder of the psychiatric hospital I had worked in many years before: dark, grey and institutional.

Admission to St Pat's, as it is known locally, was an experience I will remember forever. After the initial form-filling and answering a seemingly endless stream of questions from the admissions officer, I was escorted to the ward. I had to say my goodbyes to Peter at reception, which I did quickly and emotionlessly, as if I was rushing off for a quick fix, and followed the nurse. I will never forget the clink of the door as it locked behind me. I felt like all I was missing were the handcuffs. Jesus, it was scary.

The wards were clean but old-fashioned, as this was an old hospital which had served the public for many years. I was escorted to a bed in a six-bedded ward, where my daywear was taken away from me, my personal belongings were thoroughly searched and I was told I was strictly confined to bed in this locked ward. I felt absolutely terrified again: afraid of what was going to happen next and fearful of the other inmates, of all the strange noises and odd behaviours that were taking place around me. I was alone, all alone: without my baby, my other kids, my husband, my parents. This was new psychological pain added to what already existed: the pain of separation created excruciating and mind-blowing anguish. Was the baby being fed? Was she in a wet nappy? Was she asleep? Was she missing me, or even crying for me? All these questions were coming fast and furious into my mind. I even questioned whether God existed at all and, if he did, what was restraining his compassion towards me? *Where is he now, in my hour of need?* I wondered. 'God, this is getting more terrifying,' I cried. 'Why are you doing this to me?'

Even though I had worked in a psychiatric hospital as part of my general nurse training, I had forgotten that this was part of the routine. I had forgotten that I was sick. After all, I was now a patient, on the other side of the fence, as it were, and 'wearing a very different hat'. I can reconcile this now in some fashion as I know that the routine of this admission was for my personal safety. But at that time I felt entirely stripped of my dignity, and more like a prisoner than a patient. I remember wondering on my first very dark night there if I had mistakenly been taken to an institution for offenders, as opposed to St Patrick's Hospital. When the nurse came to administer my medication, I wondered if she was about to poison me. As she stood over me while I swallowed the tablet, I felt petrified. *Would I ever waken up again?* I thought.

Whether an explanation took place or not, I do not remember any being given. It was probably just 'a routine admission' for the staff. I feel sure this was the way that most psychiatric hospitals operated back then.

I must say, however, that most of the staff nurses were excellent: so compassionate and understanding, but certainly working within an archaic system. In an attempt to lift my mood, Peter had booked a holiday to Spain for the entire family during the Easter school holidays, but of course this was now impossible as I was in hospital, and would not be released to travel. Some of the nurses found out about the planned and now cancelled holiday. Showing so much compassion, they went out of their way to help me make special Easter baskets as a surprise for the children. Some even went out of the hospital and shopped in town during their off-duty time for little special bits to add to these baskets. I owe a sincere debt of gratitude to those nurses for their thoughtfulness and kindness, and for the real empathy for which Irish nurses have been renowned worldwide.

This made the Easter Sunday visit a very special, unexpected event for the children, although a poor second place to the holiday that they had been promised, and were so looking forward to.

In the outside world, friends knew that I was sick, but few were told where I was, or the nature of my illness. Such was the 'numbness' taking place in my family. Local gossip is always prized, and can do more to knock you down than pull you up. Peter, being well aware of this, was fearful of such gossip, and even more fearful that it would affect my business. He maintained an uncomfortable silence in an attempt to protect me. I think he had reached the end of his own coping skills. Additionally, he had to contend with finding replacement staff to keep the clinic running in my absence, which was new territory for him.

My appointed psychiatrist perscribed antidepressant medication, which I duly commenced. I reacted badly to this. Physically, it caused severe bowel problems. After several days, it was decided that I would be transferred to St James's Hospital for medical investigations. Peter accompanied me for the consultation. After preliminary examinations, it was suggested that I required emergency bowel surgery, probably an ileostomy (bowel surgery with a stoma bag). In view of the 'complex' surgery I was said to have sustained at the hands of Dr Neary, Peter suggested to the doctor we were consulting that he first call Dr Neary to get exact details. As Neary had said to me in the past: I was 'a mess'. The doctor concurred with this request.

After a short time, the doctor returned, having spoken by telephone with Neary. He said: 'Forget surgery, you are too complicated already.' I was returned to St Pat's later that day, without having received any treatment. Whatever that phone conversation with Neary entailed, I will never know, but it certainly altered the treatment protocol that the doctor had in mind.

Of course, the bowel problems were caused by side effects from medication, and was partially resolved when I was put on to a new drug. There were many changes of antidepressant drugs to follow but none were making any real difference.

After a week of confined bed rest, I was allowed up to the sitting-room area but it was still in a locked ward. Here, people sat quietly, often rocking, in varying states of *compos mentis*, without speaking and with much crying and wailing. When I had periods of sleeplessness at night, I too would go there – to pray. Many patients would remain there, rocking, smoking, crying, just like in the daytime. Very few spoke to each other: such is the nature of mental illness, I suppose. Doctors would pass in and out through the locked doors, seemingly unaware of the wails and cries, or even noticing our presence. There was either a disconnect or a familiarity, which had somehow made everything become acceptable to them.

Everything was regimented. At mealtimes, you sat at a certain table in a certain allocated position once you had been allowed out of bed. Patients were weighed at a certain time, and went to occupational workshops with military regularity. The dignity of getting one's clothes back took on a new significance.

Occupational workshops began, for me, a few weeks after I moved out to a non-locked ward. There I made trays, sugán chairs just like my dad used to make, and other small crafts. It passed the time in an otherwise very long, dull day. After another few weeks I was given a single room, which was an improvement. At least I was no longer kept awake at night by the cries of other patients. It also allowed a little more privacy for family visits. If I could not sleep, I could sit up undisturbed in my own room.

★

As the weeks passed, I kept asking for psychotherapy, but my doctor reassured me that this was exactly what she was giving me. She was a pleasant lady, known in hospital circles as 'Barbie' because of her gorgeous, seemingly endless wardrobe. But what she was doing, in my opinion, was not psychotherapy – rather, it was medication and a brief chat. Medication, in my experience, dulls the pain, gingerly placing a plaster over the real problem. It makes you sleepy, and fairly oblivious to where you are and what is going on in the real world. Medication alone neither addressed the underlying cause, nor offered a long-term solution.

I was not feeling any better, though I was assured 'I must be' by the staff, and one doctor in particular. If he came in and I was in bed, I was asked why. If I was reading, then the reading material was scrutinised and usually condemned. If I was on the phone, that did not seem right either. I seemingly could not win.

I remember, during my hospitalisation, that Peter was in the bank in Shercock, County Cavan, when robbers burst in and hit him over the head with a gun. All the customers were made to lie on the floor while they raided the bank. There was a lot of shouting, screaming and general mayhem, and, for him, the immense terror that he was would be killed. *Not only is Kathleen missing from the family, but now I'm in danger of being shot*, he had thought. He feared for the children at home. When he got out of the bank, he phoned me to relay his unfortunate encounter. He was in a very distressed state and I, naturally, became incredibly upset. I was out in the hospital grounds at the time but on my return to the ward I mentioned this to staff, who in turn called the doctor. I was told that she was very cross, and that he should not have told me this news, as stress was meant to be kept out of the equation while we were in there. *Well, was that not a natural reaction on his behalf?* I thought. *Who else would he talk to or turn to following such an ordeal?*

In my opinion, what hospital staff forgot was that life is both good and bad, and continued on in the real world while we were inmates. It was an institution, like all psychiatric hospitals were, and sometimes I felt that some staff were falling prey to the effects of institutionalisation.

After a few weeks, I was regularly allowed home for the weekend. This was not good, however, as it scared the life out of me. When I got out into the real world, it seemed like such an insecure place. I remember, on one of those early weekend discharges, going out onto the upstairs veranda at home and feeling like I wanted to jump; to end it all. No, I did not want to die, but I could not cope with continuing to live like that for the foreseeable future. There was no obvious end in sight. I even penned a song that weekend about my experience. My only fear, in jumping, was that I might not die – that I would be permanently disabled, and I could not live with any further pain. That is what really stopped me jumping.

My family would be much better off without me, I thought. *They could get on with living, rather than having this 'mad' mother who was in and out of their lives and whose moods were constantly on a swing, and who upset the entire family home.*

But I was too afraid to jump lest I become further hurt or disabled, which I knew I could not cope with, and so I returned to the incarceration of St Pat's.

I thank God daily that I did not take that plunge, and think about how much of my life with my beautiful family I would have missed out on. Suicide is *never* a solution, but I feel that can understand it, in a way, as I came as close to it as I ever hope, on that day. I also realise that I would have made headlines in the local paper that week, but I would not have been around to read about it. Rather, my family would have been condemned to living with the shame of that utter tragedy. My death would have destroyed them beyond belief.

Having been in hospital now for twelve weeks, Peter felt that I might have a better chance of recovery at home as there was no mention of me *ever* being discharged. He could see that I was not getting better in hospital. So he signed me out to go on a pilgrimage to Lourdes. I went to Lourdes with him, but cried most of the time. I was in severe panic, and fearful: fearful of what, I do not know. I felt no better than when I had first been admitted to St Pat's the year before.

I returned to St Pat's on an outpatient basis only, for a further year. On my last outpatient visit (I had chosen it as my last), my doctor there suggested changing the medication again. None of the antidepressant medicines I had taken had made the slightest improvement in my mood, or my general state of mind. Instead, I seemed to have developed many different side effects from various treatments. I pretended to gratefully accept the prescription, but on my way out I tore it up and put it in the bin. I had given fifteen months of my life to allopathic medication, and it had not worked for me, so now, I felt, it was time to change track.

Intuitively, I knew the doctors were on the wrong path with me: I was not suffering from chemical depression or even postnatal depression, but rather from post-traumatic stress. I had been incessantly researching my condition. Instinctively, I knew that medication was not going to 'fix' me – ever.

Nevertheless, postnatal depression can occur any time within a year of giving birth, so the professionals felt sure that this was the problem. (I will cover post-traumatic stress in the next chapter.)

Late that summer I made a very slow return to work, but the panic attacks continued. I was barely physically functional, but my choices were limited. Either I could lie down under this 'monster', or I could try to rise above it a little each day. I timidly chose the latter. There's a chance that, had Peter had a steady job and income, I may well have chosen the former option. I would have probably lain down under it, and would still be no further on, all these years later.

As I gradually returned to work at the clinic, a strange disconnect emerged: I could pretty much switch to a different mindset while at work. I became so immersed in my clients that I did not have time to think of my personal issues. The biggest conflict was between self-esteem and self-confidence. Self-esteem was how I felt about myself as a person and my state of being: basically, my inner environment. Self-confidence, on the other hand, was about how I related to others and external situations, and about how I utilised my particular attributes in the world at large: that was my outer environment. In other words, I was good at 'wearing the mask'. But privately, my emotions were all over the place, like sheep without a shepherd. Externally, I was confident, while internally I was like a broken glass. This was nothing new, only now my emotions were going to new heights or new depths at the wrong times, steadfastly refusing to be gathered into the fold of reason in my private moments.

Prior to my illness, I had been a confident motorist; distance did not faze me when I needed to go somewhere. Suddenly, though, I found that I could not cope with being behind the wheel of a car, and began to panic when driving. I could not overtake any vehicle, even a bicycle. Even driving at a slow speed, in my panic I felt like I was doing ten times that speed. The first time this happened was following my final release from hospital. I was driving into Monaghan to conduct a job interview for a new member of staff, and came up behind an old tractor. I was going ten miles per hour, according to my speedometer. But I felt sure that I was in a racing car at high speed, completely out of control. I absolutely could not overtake that tractor, so I had to pull over. I was shaking so badly that I had to call Peter to come and get me. That is one interview I will never forget, as I shook like a leaf in a gale-force wind. After that episode, I refused to get into the driver's seat at all for several years.

For some reason, the local church was a particularly bad place for me. Panic would set in immediately when I entered. This still baffles me. My faith in God is very strong, so why was God's house so daunting? Other churches, while not great, were inexplicably less scary; maybe I felt that I could exit more anonymously. Our local church had a tiled floor so I would have to remove my shoes on entering the back row, otherwise it was tap-tap-tap, panic-panic-panic. Getting into the queue for Holy Communion was also impossible.

I could not shop alone as I was too afraid, but my family constantly tried to encourage me to go out with them. Along with Peter, they would organise various outings under the pretence that they needed to go somewhere. I remember once going up the escalator in the Square Shopping Centre in Tallaght with Peter and the kids. It was Christmas 1997, and the centre was very busy, crowded with Christmas shoppers. As I went up the escalator I almost knocked a lady over in my panic to get off. I felt very fearful in the crowd, and decided that we had to leave – I got out of there quickly. I felt very threatened; it was all too daunting. We had scarcely been there fifteen minutes, but I could not cope with being confined. As we returned to the escalator to descend, I physically could not get on. I stood there, looking down. I was shaking and felt helpless. I visualised it as being a cable car over a deep ravine. After a long time, and much persuasion, Peter and the older children held me, and convinced me to get onto the escalator and descend backwards. When they got me to the car it was snowing outside, but on the way home we had to drive for several miles with the window rolled down as I was perspiring so profusely.

Queues anywhere were a no-go for me, so the bank, shops or any such places were impossible for me to enter. I was like a prisoner in my own body. Fear was locked inside of me, and I was always full of unknown trepidation. I was desperate, and this 'monster' was inexplicable.

Thus began my search for answers through alternative and holistic medicine. I contacted one of my former lecturers in Cheshire who was a kinesiologist of long-standing repute. He was now in his eighties, and I went to Cheshire to see him on numerous occasions. His treatment would work for me, but with the relief only lasting for a very short time. It also proved too expensive going back and forth to England, and always having to have a companion, doubling the expense. After this I went to a faith healer in Castlebar on three occasions, which did not help at all. In hindsight, his work seemed the height of quackery. I went to a hypnotherapist I had heard of, but would only get a short-term reprieve from my symptoms. I also consulted a Chinese acupuncturist in Dublin for numerous sessions, with no benefit.

Meanwhile, I was doing all sorts of nutritional and alternative programs. I could not afford to be ill, but equally I could not afford these programmes, as they were costing my family money that we did not have. We were broke, but I felt that I had no choice, as I was desperate to get well. So, as I worked and earned, I paid for more and more therapy and treatment. Every cent seemed to go towards therapy of some sort.

I then consulted a colleague working as a hypnotherapist, who got me back driving, but I could still only manage to drive locally. To this day, driving into cities or areas of heavy traffic is not for me. The hypnotherapist could not address that unrelenting fear and panic, so he referred me to a psychotherapist. I attended sessions with this doctor for eighteen months, but had to stop due to the cost and lack of any real and lasting progress. Following this, I found Dr Michael Corry, a holistic psychiatrist, whom I attended at Clane Hospital. He was the man who instantly diagnosed the real cause of my problem, the truth: that I was suffering from post-traumatic stress syndrome. For financial reasons, I could not attend him as often as was required, in his opinion. Then, sadly, he died at a young age.

Still on my quest for a cure, I enrolled as a student of naturopathy and herbalism at Griffith College, Dublin, in 2000. I was desperately trying to find answers to my continuing ill health. At Griffith College I learned a great deal, gained a distinction diploma qualification in herbalism and naturopathy, and made some amazing friends. I received support, compassion and understanding, both from my lecturers and classmates. My classmates brought me to the realisation that I was brutally wronged, unnecessarily scared, and needed to see justice done. They encouraged me to continue fighting for answers and for justice. For the support I received from my lecturers and fellow students, I am eternally grateful.

Through the intervening years, I was constantly seeking help from other holistic health sources. Were it not for my wonderful colleagues in the clinic, I feel sure that I would not have made it. When I was down and they could see it, they gently coaxed me into undergoing more intensive therapy, but they were never forceful, as they recognised my fragility. When I was up, they celebrated with me. Much of the therapy they afforded me was free of charge. My colleagues put together packages of reflexology, physical therapy, osteopathy, acupuncture, hypnotherapy, cranial fluid dynamics and nutritional and herbal programmes, which gradually pushed me up the ladder of life. I am proud to say that my team are chosen from the best available. I feel absolutely sure that I have hand-picked not just the best team for my clients, but for me personally in my quest for wellness. They have become like an extension of my own family. Many of them have worked with me for the past twenty years. To all of my colleagues, I owe a huge debt of gratitude. I want to say thank you, from the bottom of my heart. You may never know how you have saved and retrieved my broken life: so, *mile buiochas*.

★

I can now see clearly how a person can become locked into the revolving-door system, being repeatedly admitted to a psychiatric institution due to a lack of satisfactory progress in their outside-of-the-institution programme, even with frequently offered alterations to medication. This can happen especially if one does not have the knowledge, skill or support to think outside the medical model. It would be easy to become so institutionalised that you could become fearful of living in the outside world, once you become accustomed to the militaristic regime and false security that exists within those grey walls. Fear can become a serious emotion: it might seem safer to stay inside and be medicated than to face the real world in a quest for wellness.

In my opinion, this is where the wider fears surrounding mental illness are born. In the past, people knew that the risk of institutional incarceration was a very real thing, so it was better to suffer in silence than to be abandoned by family, who, in many cases, might never see them again, if the sufferer was institutionalised.

Psychiatric units serve many people, but I feel that their care only treats half the problem. Medication dulls the symptoms, but the underlying cause – for which there is *always* a trigger – does not appear to feature much in treatment. In my experience, both from working in the psychiatric service and from being a patient, medication alone is never enough. Every patient with mental-health issues has a story to tell, a cause and a starting point to relate, if they are really deeply listened to. Changing medication is just not enough. Has much really changed in that field, to this day?

Medication without 'talk therapy' to help the underlying cause is never an answer. Of course, some people definitely need medication during this period – that is indisputable. For any readers currently taking such medication, it would be grossly irresponsible to discontinue it without the supervision of your doctor. But do not let that stop you from seeking other answers through therapy. Properly structured talk therapy needs to co-exist alongside medication, if such is warranted in the short term, and is a current short-term working solution for the individual. The only thing we all have in common is that we are all different, with a certain amount of necessary conformity enabling us to coexist within society. But society has tried to press us into the same mould, to homogenise us, since the dawn of time. There is no one size that fits all. Each person's story is different, and psychiatric and mental health programmes need to be individually tailored, with 'talk therapy' being instituted at some point. It is stating the obvious that each person is unique, but it means that each person's programme must, equally, be uniquely tailored to them.

We are constantly surrounded by sadness, melancholy or depression. The reality is that there is no generation, or stratum of society, in Ireland that hasn't, at some point, been touched by this. Success is achieved by successfully managing the bumps in the road, and maintaining one's sanity. Otherwise, we could all be in that perpetually revolving door of psychiatry, where hope quickly slips away each time we enter into it.

★

When I worked in psychiatry in Monaghan, in 1978, a leading

psychiatrist there, Dr John Owens, was a pioneer in opening up mental hospitals into the community. His premise was that he would get people back into the communities where they belonged. He was a great believer in breaking down those high grey walls, getting patients out rather than in. With tremendous foresight, he initiated a now-current system. But the wheels of change moved very slowly indeed.

In 1996, we were still living in 'old Ireland', where you could acceptably have any kind of illness except mental illness. Change to such entrenched attitudes comes slowly, and the movement was still only in its infancy.

On one of my weekend discharges from hospital, I remember my eldest daughter taking a phone call one night. When she did not return to the sitting room after I heard her hang up the phone, I went to investigate, only to find her in floods of tears. At first she did not want to tell me what had happened, but eventually she admitted that a lady (later a client) had called and asked if it was true that I had slit my wrists. Imagine asking a fourteen-year-old child that question about her own mother, a child who didn't fully understand what that meant, what was really happening in her life or why her family was broken. I had never slit my wrists, but I was disturbed by the malice of that phone call on many levels. Ironically, it seems that that lady needed me before I needed her.

That is the way that mental health has been treated and interpreted in the past. There was a great stigma attached to any mental-health issues in Ireland at that time, especially in relationto psychiatric-hospital admissions.

We have had apologies from governments in this country over

various abuses, but never for the cruel incarcerations, over decades, in mental institutions which were, to say the least, archaic. This was, in my opinion, a harkening back to the days of mass institutionalisation and incarceration of so many people in psychiatric hospitals, with inmates often being subjected to living out their final days in these institutions. It appears to me that certain people were not necessarily mentally ill: unmarried mothers, for example, were often amongst those long-term admissions. Some were people who had unfortunately fallen on hard times, and got 'down' in themselves. But they were not all insane. Surely it was criminal behaviour on behalf of the professionals who kept them there, and perhaps even a subject warranting future investigation.

Psychiatric institutions were the forgotten hospitals housing a forgotten people, walled off from society, where individuals were housed in large, dark, grey, daunting buildings, where families visited rarely, if at all. So many people were hospitalised within these grey walls for their entire lives. Families often never again spoke about their 'missing' relatives, and might see their institutionalisation as a slight upon themselves and their families. Who was really at fault here for their long-term removal from their homes? Why did this happen, and why was it allowed to continue for so long?

When I was a student working in the psychiatric division in 1978, one ward sister christened me 'the Rebel'. I disputed the system of psychiatric treatment back then in 1977, as I saw patients being medicated and disciplined but never really listened to or spoken to as adults or human beings. Everything had a time, and routine was important 'for the staff'. Of course, many people had been inpatients at the hospital for several years, abandoned in shame by their families, with no voice and no means of release. Some even became mute on entering such places. Often, they were reduced to being put in 'the dungeon' or 'black hole' as it was called, for their repeated requests for a cigarette. There was little or no formal activity, and no occupational therapy during the day, so they mostly sat and rocked themselves. This in itself would depress the most sane people. Some staff were only identifiable by their uniforms; the longer they worked there, the more institutionalised they became. Surely this is inhumane and wrong, irrespective of the century we live in.

This culture has, thankfully, changed, with many patients now being treated in their own communities. People suffering from long-term mental-health incapacities, and requiring full-time care, are now housed in more 'home-like' situations, usually based in the annex of the hospital or within their community – which is wonderful. Of course, mental-health issues are still an ongoing part of life and will always be with us, so we do not want the pendulum to swing too far in the opposite direction, where sufferers cannot access inpatient care if it is necessary for their immediate safety. In about 1978, some forward-thinking psychiatrists, like Dr Owens in Ireland, started looking at alternative ways of treating mental-health issues in the wider community. But much more remains to be done, especially about the high suicide rate. These unfortunate people are slipping through the net somewhere, and need to be identified early, and helped. There is much talk about the Irish culture of alcohol abuse: I wonder if that is their 'ism', temporarily giving them time out. Perhaps this could be a cue from which to begin.

Is it that psychiatrists in the past had got used to the 'same old, same old', or that they had a fear of moving or thinking outside of the norm, and listening to their clients?

Is that still missing?

Chapter 7
Post-traumatic Stress Disorder

So what is this 'monstrous' condition called post-traumatic stress disorder? I will refer to this condition from here on in as PTSD.

Many papers and articles have been written over the years about PTSD. For the past nineteen years, I have researched and scrutinised much of what has been collated by various experts, in an attempt to understand what it is all about. My interest, of course, was in gaining insight into what was going on in my own emotions.

PTSD has in the past been called 'shell shock', 'battle-fatigue syndrome' or 'war neurosis', because of its prevalence among war veterans returning from various wars. It is a lasting consequence of traumatic experiences.

The British National Institute of Mental Health describes it as 'a condition that develops after a terrifying ordeal'. An army veteran of the Iraq war wrote in *The New York Times Magazine* in May 2014:

Post-traumatic stress disorder can be treated, but it never goes away. On bad days, this condition is so close, you cannot breathe. On good days, it is off in the distance like a gathering storm, whose cold wind only just touches your neck.

This is a frightening prospect, for someone trying to recover.

If, at any time in their life, an individual senses that they are in danger, it is natural to feel afraid. This fear, however, triggers many split-second changes in the body as a defence mechanism against danger, or in an attempt to avoid it. This is called the 'fear-fight-flight' response, and is a healthy reaction that protects the individual from harm. When your senses of safety and trust are shattered, it is normal to feel unhinged, numb and disconnected, to experience nightmares and to fear and dwell upon the event for some time. It is a normal reaction to abnormal events. These symptoms, however, are in most cases short-lived.

PTSD can develop following a horrific or terrifyingly traumatic event, which threatens someone's safety or makes them feel helpless. The fear-fight-flight reaction is warped or damaged, leaving the sufferer feeling stressed or frightened, even when the danger no longer exists. The traumatic event is usually so overwhelming and frightening that it would upset any individual.

With PTSD, the symptoms do not decrease, and you do not feel a little better each day. In fact, the symptoms may start to increase, leaving the afflicted person feeling worse and worse. PTSD is a mental-health disorder where mind and body remain in ongoing shock. There is a major disconnect between your memory of the event and your feelings about it. This results when the traumatic event causes an over-reactive adrenaline response, creating deep neurological patterns of change in the brain. Studies put the likelihood of PTSD among women who experience a traumatic birth at 2 percent.

The intensity of PTSD revolves around the nature of the traumatic event, and has been found to be more serious when the event involves the perception of a severe threat to your life or personal safety. The more extreme and intense the threat, the greater the risk there is of developing PTSD as a response. Intentionally inflicted harm, from another human, tends to have a more traumatic effect on a person, leaving them with a higher risk of developing PTSD, than 'acts of God', such as natural disasters. The extent to which the traumatic event was unexpected, uncontrollable and inescapable, plays a role in the severity of the PTSD experienced, and the ability – or inability – of the individual to recover from it.

Three main symptoms of PTSD have been identified:

1. Reliving the traumatic event.
2. Avoiding reminders of the event.
3. Increased anxiety and emotional arousal.

1. Re-experiencing the trauma includes what I call the 'link and connect' symptoms and reactions to the initial trauma:

- Upsetting and intrusive memories of the event, with the sufferer constantly reliving the ordeal through thoughts and memories.
- Flashbacks, as if the event were happening over and over again.
- Nightmares of the event, or fearful dreams.
- Feeling intensely distressed when reminded of the trauma.

- Intense physical reactions when reminded of the event. These may include rapid breathing, pounding heart, sweating, nausea, fainting, muscular tension and a feeling of 'going to pieces'. Such triggers may include reading media articles or seeing a television reminder of the initial setting, event, or person involved. They can start from the person's own thoughts and feelings. Words, objects or situations which are reminders of the event can also trigger a re-experiencing of the event.

2. Avoiding reminders of the trauma:

- Avoiding stimuli that remind you of the event. This may include people, thoughts, events, places, feelings or anniversaries. This leads to significant disruption in a person's daily living, affecting every aspect including social, occupational, sexual and family life.
- Unable to remember important aspects of the trauma.
- Loss of general interest in life and normal activities.
- Feeling emotionally numb.
- Strong feelings of guilt, depression or worry that are unrelenting.
- Sexual dysfunction and lack of interest in sex.
- Feeling detached from reality and family.
- Feeling you have no future on this earth.

3. Increased anxiety and emotional arousal:

- Feeling easily startled and jumpy or nervous.
- Sleep difficulties: difficulties falling asleep, or staying asleep, dream-disturbed sleep and generally wakening unrefreshed following a reasonable amount of sleep.
- Unprovoked angry outbursts, or ongoing irritability.
- Poor concentration.
- Always on 'red alert', always on the edge and ready to run, always in fear-fight-flight mode.
- Guilt and self-blame.
- Shame.
- Mistrust and feelings of betrayal.
- Problems relating to others or difficulty showing affection.
- Depression and a feeling of hopelessness.
- Thoughts or actions of suicide or self-harm, including attempted suicide.
- Feeling alone and alienated.
- Physical symptoms like aches and pains, increased blood pressure and heart rate, rapid breathing, muscle tension, nausea, diarrhoea, appetite changes, weight changes.
- Substance abuse, which may include cigarettes, alcohol and drugs, including abuse of prescription medication.

PTSD can affect those who personally experience the catastrophe, those who witness it or those who pick up the pieces afterwards. It may extend to emergency workers, law enforcement officers or the friends and family of those who went through the trauma. It may differ from person to person. It can occur within hours of the event, or it can be several years before symptoms appear, but it typically emerges after a delay of at least thirty days. Most of the PTSD sufferers that we hear about are battle-scarred soldiers since the condition achieved prominence in the 1980s in the wake of the trauma reported by American survivors of the Vietnam war. In fact, about 7.7 million Americans are affected by this condition. But it goes well beyond American soldiers: it extends to all areas and people. Any overwhelming life experience which at least involves a risk of serious injury, death or loss of physical integrity can trigger PTSD, especially if the event feels unpredictable and uncontrollable. The response to this event involves intense fear, horror or helplessness. Events triggering this might include rape, mugging, kidnap, torture, child abuse, natural disasters or medical misadventure.

Diagnosis is largely symptom-based, with criteria defined for the severity of the condition, as the course of the illness may vary. Some people recover within six months, while others live out their lives as PTSD sufferers.

The Diagnostic and Statistical Manual of Mental Disorders IV summarises the criteria as:

A. Exposure to a traumatic event involving loss of 'physical integrity', risk of serious personal injury or death to self or others, 'outside the range of usual human experience'.

B. Persistent re-experiencing or intense negative psychological or physiological responses to any objective or subjective reminder of the traumatic event.

C. Persistent avoidance and emotional numbing.

D. Persistent symptoms of increased arousal not present before the event.

E. Duration of symptoms for more than one month.

F. Significant impairment or distress in life activities or important areas of normal daily functioning.

To move on, it is very important to 'face' and 'feel your emotions and memories. Effective treatment does exist. We must attempt to embrace the pain and burn it as fuel for our journey.

PTSD is not a sign of weakness. The only way to overcome it is to confront what happened by learning to accept it as part of your past, and as part of life's journey. I hasten to add that I do not wish to minimise the event you or I have experienced.

Avoidance of, or failure to confront, your pain will ultimately harm you, your relationships, your ability to function, your general quality of life and your health. It can even destroy you. The best way to get rid of the pain is to feel the pain. When you feel the pain and go beyond it, you will find an intense love waiting to be awakened within yourself. There is nothing enlightening about shrinking, so other people will not feel insecure around you. As we are liberated from our fear, our presence automatically liberates others. Grief is not evil or some kind of disease. It is a normal part of healthy living, a safety valve for us to use in times of loss. We must give ourselves permission to shout and cry for as long as it takes to get through it, and find relative peace at the other end. The crying will stop when the crying is finished. There will of course be very bad days, but we must avoid those well-meaning but often dangerous people who think that our bad days and our problems are the result of a Valium deficiency. I feel like they must either live in ignorance, or have something to gain from their devious misunderstanding.

For many years I entertained the notion that I had become 'complex and analytical' after my life-changing trauma in 1995. But on reflection, delving through various scraps I have written over the past nineteen years, I realise that I was searching, and reflecting deeply on the importance of spirituality in my life. Whenever I felt uncomfortable in my own skin – which was often – I used to look left and right, before and after, to see who or what was causing it. I always knew who the principal culprit was, but this knowledge never made any difference to how I felt. Now, when I feel uncomfortable in my skin, I look at my own attitudes, and it always makes a difference for the better. Neary's actions had me under siege: overwhelmed and crushed. They assumed control over my life for nineteen years. This was more than half of my entire married life. I thank God I can now see things differently – most of the time.

Psychological treatment allows you to:

- Explore your feelings and thoughts.
- Work through negative emotions.
- Learn how to cope with the intrusive memories.
- Address some of the issues PTSD has caused in your life and relationships.

Examples of treatments available include:

- Psychotherapy (what I call 'talk therapy') conducted with a mental-health or other qualified professional, which may either be on a one-to-one basis or in a group setting, or occasionally both. The intention of talk therapy is to teach the person helpful ways to react to frightening events that trigger their PTSD symptoms, as part of their ultimate quest for healing.

- Cognitive behavioural therapy is especially valuable. It has an emphasis on feared stimuli. This therapy looks at triggers such as thoughts, feelings or situations reminding you of the event. It acts by changing your patterns of thinking and the behaviour responsible for negative emotions. True, nobody can ever change the events that have happened, but they can help you alter how you are coping, or not coping, in the wake of those painful events.

- EMDR (eye movement, de-sensitisation and reprocessing therapy). This is a form of psychotherapy and involves elements of cognitive behavioural therapy combined with voluntary rapid-eye movements, where the person concentrates on memories, feelings or thoughts of the trauma. It is intended to 'unfreeze' the brain's information-processing system, which has been interrupted in times of extreme stress.

- Cranial-fluid dynamics is based on an American model of ontological medicine. It is conducted using a combination of kinesiology and associated hand modes. This helps break traits held in the subconscious brain, with a deep healing effect – breaking chains, as it were. This can assist the sufferer in moving forward in their life, with only a distant memory of the traumatic event remaining.

- Family therapy is a valuable tool, as the entire family can be injured from the effects of this condition. It can help the affected family to understand what the sufferer is going through, as well as helping them through their own dilemmas. When one family member is affected by such a sudden and severe condition, the entire family unit can be thrown into crisis. In my opinion, family therapy is not as widely offered in Ireland as it should be.

- Prescribed medication may, in some instances, be necessary. But while it may have adjunctive benefit, it does not always treat the underlying cause. Because it may temporarily make the person feel better as they are less sad, anxious or depressed, it has, in my opinion, limited benefit as a curative tool unless used in tandem with other therapies. For some sufferers, medication can be so much of a crutch as to become an addiction, adding an extra dimension to their existing problems. This may serve only to exacerbate their problems rather than heal them.

- Regular moderate exercise positively impacts on the physical and psychological well-being of all individuals. Exercise increases endorphins, the 'happy hormones' in the body, which can only be beneficial in uplifting the spirit of the sufferer. Additionally, in PTSD sufferers, it serves as a distraction from disturbing emotions, raises self-esteem and gives a feeling of control. Unfortunately, the PTSD sufferer often lacks the motivation to exercise regularly due to the inconsistency of the emotional condition. It is easier to find twenty reasons not to exercise than to find one that is truly valuable.

- Finally, I would add that, for PTSD, there is no one treatment that cures all sufferers. Rather than one, a collection of therapies may be needed to break the relentless cycle of trauma and release the sufferer into a place of relative freedom.

In conclusion, some important things for PTSD sufferers to remember are:

- Reach out to others for support in an attempt to ease your disconnect with society. This is not always easy, and involves moving out of your comfort zone little by little.

- Avoid alcohol and self-medicating, either with prescription or over-the-counter drugs. This may only serve to compound your problems and make you feel worse in the long run.

- Challenge your sense of helplessness, as trauma leaves you feeling powerless and vulnerable.

- Spend time out in nature, either with family or as a member of a local organisation that offers outdoor recreation or team-building opportunities.

- Family members of a PTSD sufferer need to pay special attention to their own self-care, and to avail of any eavailable extra support. PTSD takes a very heavy toll on the entire family; it can be difficult for them to understand the condition as they have been cast into this situation suddenly and unexpectedly. But if the caregiver falls down, so too does the sufferer.

Chapter 8
Neary Scandal Exposed

It was a pleasant autumn morning in October 1998. As I peered through the kitchen window, I could see the trees beginning to shed their leaves in the October breeze. In keeping with my routine, I had dragged myself out of bed before 6 AM to pray for an hour in the quiet of the morning. Keeping abreast with household chores before awakening the children for school, I was doing my usual early morning ironing, listening to the television in the background. The seven o'clock news came on TV3 with the announcement of a journalistic bombshell:

> Dr Michael Neary, consultant obstetrician at Our Lady of Lourdes Hospital, Drogheda, has been placed on administrative leave having been suspected of performing multiple unnecessary caesarean hysterectomies.
>
> News of this allegation was released to media by the North-Eastern Health Board.

As if I had been struck by lightning, I froze and felt stuck to where I was standing. I was in a state of awe and disbelief. The iron dropped out of my hand and smashed onto the floor. I tried to shout for Peter, but my voice was so faint that it carried only as a whisper. Hearing the thud of the iron, Peter came running, thinking I had fainted. He said I was deathly white, and pulled a chair over to sit me down. He was in panic mode, shouting, 'What happened? What happened?' The children had heard the commotion and my eldest daughter, then aged sixteen, came dashing into the kitchen with Rescue Remedy, well aware that there might be another crisis. (Rescue Remedy is a Dr Bach flower formula used for shock and distress, and its use had become the new norm in our house since my trauma in 1995.)

I had once again imploded. My thoughts and emotions were every which way. I had gone from feeling reasonably good a few minutes earlier, to feeling bad, to in between, to feeling that I was going mad. All of this had happened within seconds, at a frightening pace. Initially I thought they must have got the doctor's name incorrect. I was suspicious of another consultant working at the same hospital. I was, after all, still a staunch believer in Neary. I had hoped and trusted that he had told me the whole truth, and had worked in my best interests, as any doctor would, and was not guided by a personal, twisted agenda in his actions on 10 July 1995. Such was the range of thoughts rushing through my mind.

I had worked with this man. I had employed and paid him to deliver a level of quality and safe care. Surely he was honest and honourable enough to have given me that? *Is it? It couldn't be, but maybe it's real. Oh my God, am I going mad?* Such was my range of jostled thoughts, as I continued to feel faint. By now, every window in our kitchen had been flung wide open. I remember sweating profusely.

This overwhelming reaction meant that I had to cancel seeing clients that day. I felt like I was only barely clinging on to life.

Cancelling clients had become a familiar theme over the past three years, but work was the last thing I needed or could think of at that moment. My family took care of that, as I was unable to think clearly, after that announcement on TV3.

A chill crept over me, and a feeling of malaise. Beads of perspiration began to trickle down my brow, over my eyelids and into my eyes. It felt like acid was burning my eyes, causing me to blink rapidly. As they inched me back to bed, Peter and Arlene either holding me up or dragging me, I was crying profusely. This was one of the worst disasters that could befall me. Once more the entire household was in turmoil because of me, as I had crashed once more. What an emotional state to send the children out to school in: upset and stressed, not understanding what this crisis was all about. The children were once again terrified. *Why was I such a bad mother?* I thought. This was all my fault, surely. *Why can't I cope?* Guilt kept hitting me like I was being dashed off rocks.

My three-year-old daughter, Caoimhe, climbed into the bed beside me. As she snuggled into my chest, she repeatedly told me, 'It will be okay, Mammy.' But I could not see that. Neither she nor I understood what 'it' was. I cried and cried, my tears leaving her soft black curls saturated. The news that morning had the effect of reinforcing my panic. I felt helpless, not knowing who or where to turn to for further help or information.

I lay in bed that day, curtains tightly closed, full of trepidation. As the morning progressed, scant details kept appearing in each ensuing news bulletin, but no concrete information was forthcoming. My mother phoned several times after she heard the news, knowing only too well the detrimental effect that this news would have on her little girl. Like any parent, she was worried about her child, yet feeling helpless to make things better, to make it go away. She knew all too well how fragile my nervous system was, and that I was closely skirting another breakdown, even without this news. She feared that this could push me over the edge, and dreaded the possibility of me returning to a psychiatric institution. In short, Mom was in a state of despair, and several hundred miles away. I was back in the grip of a relentless fear. This latest setback kept me out of work for several days.

★

At this juncture, I would like to outline how this information was exposed, and the multiple inquiries which followed the exposure.

This revelation came about due to the tremendous bravery of two midwives who had trained in another hospital, and had gone to work as staff midwives at the Lourdes Hospital. In late October 1998, during a meeting with North-Eastern Health Board officials on a separate matter, they raised their concerns to the board's lawyer. They stated that they felt alarmed by the hysterectomy rate and what they saw as the dubious practices of Neary at the Lourdes Hospital.

The lawyer and his associates should be applauded for neither turning a blind eye nor a deaf ear to the allegations. Rather, following the conclusion of that meeting, the lawyer called the human resources director, who in turn called the clinical director and the deputy chief executive of the North-Eastern Health Board.

What ensued immediately was a preliminary check of medical records at the Lourdes Hospital Maternity Unit, which, frighteningly, confirmed the Health Board's suspicions. Dr Neary was abroad at the time, but was duly informed of the complaints made against him, and he denied everything.

I applaud these midwives' courage as, despite receiving a number of threatening notes and phone calls – and even death threats, as has been reported by the media – they bravely held to their concerns and continued with their allegations, exposing the bizarre obstetric practices at the Lourdes Hospital.

We repeatedly hear governments vouch for and encourage whistleblowers, but in reality we know it is often very different when it happens. They are often vilified by colleagues, as they have rattled the status quo. Instead of being lauded for their bravery, they too have become victims, and their lives are changed irreversibly.

Has much changed to this day? It appears that the notion of whistleblowing is wonderful in theory, but not always in practice.

In light of the concerns raised by these midwives, the North-Eastern Health Board had no choice but to request that Neary take two weeks' administrative leave from his post as a consultant obstetrician-gynaecologist at the hospital. Meanwhile, the deputy chief executive of the North-Eastern Health Board, became more informed, and increasingly alarmed, about the incidence of peripartum hysterectomies. A peripartum hysterectomy refers to the surgical removal of the uterus or womb, during or around the time of, giving birth. This led to major misgivings about permitting Neary back to work. Neary was defiant, and continued to deny the malpractices of which he was accused. The Health Board had set out plans to take out a High Court injunction, preventing Neary from setting foot in any hospital again until an audit of his work was conducted. The more hospital charts the hospital managers examined, the greater the scandal that unfolded. They wanted to extend his suspension. It sounded to me like there must have been chaotic scenes and sleepless nights amongst Health Board officials during this time. This led to the first of many investigations.

Investigation 1: Review by the Irish Hospital Consultants Association

The Irish Hospital Consultants Association was established to promote, encourage and support the advancement of the practice of medicine in all specialties and areas, and the improvement of the health Services in Ireland. They have a membership of 2,400.

The Health Board subjected Neary's cases of caesarean hysterectomies during the period 1996 to 1998 to review, and they were audited by the Irish Hospital Consultants Association. Erroneously, or curiously, it was believed that the caesarean hysterectomy rate was within acceptable limits before 1996. Perhaps it was suspected that Dr Neary had emotionally derailed following the untimely death of his wife, Gabrielle, in 1996, leading him to perform so many hysterectomies; but this theory was later disproved. Already it was a case of his own ssociation investigating him.

The three consultant obstetrician-gynaecologists investigating were, interestingly, selected by Neary and his representative organisation. These doctors, from the Coombe Hospital and the National Maternity Hospital in Holles Street, Dublin, were highly regarded in their field at that time and called 'eminent professionals'. They were given seventeen patient files from the maternity theatre register, on women whom Neary had performed peripartum hysterectomies. Eight files were quickly ruled out of consideration as Neary claimed, the women concerned had consented to the removal of their wombs for the purpose of sterilisation, a procedure banned at the hospital until 1997. On that point alone, Neary should have been deemed out of order, as these procedures were performed while the ban existed. By performing these sterilisations, he was non-compliant with the terms of his employment and the hospital's code of conduct.

There is no available evidence that any of these three doctors either questioned or investigated his claim. They appeared to accept his declaration at face value, without querying or commenting on the hospital's code of ethics.

This left nine patient files to be examined, most of whom were very young women. The investigators, perhaps hurriedly, compiled their report, which was furnished to the Health Board by Neary's lawyers. Legal teams were shocked and dismayed by the report's findings.

Little surprise, though, that these three individuals exonerated Neary and were unanimous in their view that he should be immediately allowed to return to work at the Lourdes Hospital. This was the prevailing feeling of collegiality in that era, but that certainly did not make it right. Whether or not the association expected the North-Eastern Health Board to accept their recommendations at face value is unknown.

Based on the report of the Irish Hospital Consultants Association, Health Board officials, having sought advice, felt legally obliged to allow Neary back to work, despite profound reservations. They saw this as a serious blow, and it meant that they did not have a chance of getting the intended High Court order.

Two of the investigating obstetricians reported that:

> We are of the opinion that all of the nine cases reviewed can be justified in the prevailing situation. We find no evidence of questionable clinical judgement, poor operative ability or faulty decision-making. Quite the contrary, we find that Dr Neary in the exercise of his clinical judgement, has, under difficult circumstances, probably saved the lives of several mothers. On the evidence presented, we find no grounds to suspend Dr Neary or to place any restrictions on his public or private practice.

It is not known which two doctors were the authors of this statement. Neither do we know the identity of the third obstetrician, who enthusiastically made the following declaration about his Drogheda colleague:

> It is my firm conclusion that Dr Neary should continue to work at Our Lady of Lourdes Hospital pending any formal investigation. It would be wrong to put restrictions on his practice. It is my view that the mothers of the North-Eastern Health Board region are fortunate in having the service of such an experienced and caring obstetrician.

Dr Neary returned to work in November 1998 on the condition that he be assisted by a locum consultant for caesarean sections, and that no peripartum hysterectomies would be performed by him without first calling in another consultant. No hysterectomies were performed during this period.

This can only lead one to believe that both Neary and the hospital staff were well aware that the eyes of the nation and the world were now upon them – the news story had received both national and international media attention. Attitudes had drastically changed within the hospital, and it seemed that everybody was watching their back. Greater efforts were now being made to preserve a woman's uterus, even when faced with massive obstetric haemorrhage.

His return lasted only four weeks.

Investigation 2: Review by Dr Maresh

The deputy chief executive of the North-Eastern Health Board and his officials were not at all comfortable with the Irish Hospital Consultants report, and wisely asked for a second opinion from an obstetrician outside the jurisdiction. They chose Dr Michael Maresh from St Mary's Hospital, Manchester, England. This hospital had a birth rate of 6,000 babies per annum. Dr Maresh examined the same nine files which had been reviewed in the exoneration of Neary by the three Irish doctors. His report was never made available to the public, but much was divulged in a leak to the Irish Times, probably from an informed source within the Health Board. These leaks made their way into the media, and thus into the public domain. Further revelations of his findings were eventually divulged in Judge Harding Clark's report.

Dr Maresh confirmed the Health Board's worst fears, and expressed major concerns about what he had reviewed in the files. Dr Maresh was equally concerned about Dr Neary being permitted to continue working as a consultant obstetrician: he felt that this could put more women in his care at risk.

He asserted that Neary's clinical judgement was significantly impaired, that women were being put at risk, and that he should immediately stop practising. Dr Maresh indicated that he had concerns about other aspects of Neary's patient management, such as his skills in performing caesarean sections if and when he encountered complications. He reckoned that Neary's perception of events appeared impaired.

On the basis of this report, the North-Eastern Health Board officials felt that they had sufficient legal grounds to put Neary on immediate administrative leave, having him cease working at the hospital from 11 December 1998. Neary agreed to this, and the Irish Hospital Consultants Association backed off the case. Why this action was suddenly taken, we were never told. Dr Maresh's review had turned the original report on its head.

A more profound search of the Lourdes Hospital theatre register dating back to 1991 was conducted. This year was chosen because it was the year the current register had commenced. No mention of this search was made prior to that period. This would now lead to yet another investigation by a Review Group.

One hundred and twenty-nine women had lost their

wombs, and effectively been castrated by Neary. Many were young women with the potential to have more children. Twenty-five of them were first-time mothers. Many of those babies died in the perinatal period. He had donned God's mantle, and decided their fate.

Throughout this period, all former patients were kept in the dark as to what was happening in the investigation, the identity of patients involved in the investigation, or any other information concerning our fate. To my knowledge there was no formal communication sent from the Health Board to any ex-patient. At least, I did not receive any, nor did any of those I have asked. It was as if it was none of our business, though we were the central characters in this situation.

Chapter 9
Investigation 3: The Review Group Investigation

The North-Eastern Health Board, recommended that a Review Group be set up, following scrutiny of the Lourdes Hospital theatre register by officials. The purpose was to seek assistance and advice on review of Dr Neary's peripartum hysterectomy practice in the period between 1992 and 1998.

In response to the North-Eastern Health Board's request, Dr Harith Lamki, chairman of the Institute of Obstetricians and Gynaecologists, Royal College of Physicians of Ireland, agreed to commission the Review Group. This group consisted of three obstetricians and gynaecologists.

They held their first meeting on 6 January 1999.

Their terms of reference were:

1. To review Dr Neary's clinical practice as obstetrician and gynaecologist at Our Lady of Lourdes Hospital, Drogheda, during the said period.

2. To consider and assess the nature and merit of the concerns of the Health Board regarding the suspected high incidence of peripartum caesarean hysterectomies carried out from 1992 to 1998 by Dr Neary.

3. To report their findings to the Health Board and Dr Neary.

They studied the clinical charts of forty-two patients who had had a peripartum caesarean hysterectomy carried out during the years 1992 to 1998. Following amendments, and after agreed exclusions, the charts of thirty-nine patients were examined. Amendments were made to their review, as three of the identified hysterectomy surgeries were deemed not to have been performed by Neary.

They interviewed Dr Neary, his obstetric colleagues, anaesthetists, midwives and pathologists, as well as management personnel at the Lourdes Hospital. Notably, not a single patient concerned was contacted or interviewed by the group to get their side of the story or revisit their experience. The Review Group report was issued in April 1999.

The report was shocking, though I did not gain access to it until years later. The central victims were once again, kept in the dark. In brief, Neary had performed 708 caesarean sections and thirty-nine peripartum hysterectomies during his period of practice. They found that Neary's career peripartum caesarean hysterectomy rate was one in every twenty, which is twenty times more than that recorded in one Dublin hospital. His reasons for performing caesarean sections were also questioned as 'dubious means of delivery'. In the Dublin hospital they referred to, which is unnamed, there were only eight peripartum hysterectomies in 38,816 deliveries, which is a rate of 1:441. Between 1993 and 1998, Neary's peripartum hysterectomy rate was one in every seventeen. In the Coombe Maternity Hospital, Dublin, the rate was 1:600. Holles Street Maternity Hospital had a rate of 1:405. What a difference in practice. What made the difference, and why?

The Review Group formed the following opinions:

- In the cases of eighteen patients, Neary's decision to perform a peripartum hysterectomy was not acceptable clinical practice.

- For sixteen patients, his decision was considered 'acceptable'.

- In the remaining five cases it was deemed as 'doubtful practice'.

While severe blood loss was one of Neary's repeatedly cited reasons for performing a hysterectomy, the group found, that this was, in several cases, unjustified, as blood loss in most of these patients was not found to be excessive. His decision to perform a hysterectomy was precipitous at times, as he did not wait to see if bleeding would spontaneously cease, without risk to the patient's life. They concluded that his unexplained response to blood loss was either a 'low-tolerance threshold for bleeding' or a 'panic reaction'.

★

While Dr Neary suggested that obtaining blood for transfusion was often difficult, the Review Group considered that the amount of blood loss was frequently overestimated by him, and would therefore not have warranted a transfusion. His concerns about the ready availability of blood for transfusion were unfounded. Blood was always available within the hospital, as confirmed by laboratory pathologists. If required in unusually large amounts, additional supplies would have been readily available from the Dublin blood bank.

There was a substantial discrepancy between the recorded pathological and clinical findings. In most cases, a uterus without significant pathology was removed, as shown on histological assessment reports from the laboratory.

These findings are repugnant on many levels, in my estimation. Such invasive and life-changing surgery is traumatic for any woman, even when it is required as a life-saving measure. To unnecessarily put women through such a traumatic procedure is noxious, and surely displays criminal intent. These heinous crimes have never been adjudicated by a criminal court. There must have been some private satisfaction on Neary's part in carrying out such extensive mutilation.

The clinical diagnosis of a morbidly adherent placenta was indicated by Neary in a number of the patient charts examined. But the Review Group disputed this finding, since it was not confirmed histologically (by laboratory testing) in *almost all* of these patients. At interview, Neary blamed the pathologists for this. But, prior to being interviewed, he had never questioned pathological findings during all the years that he had worked there. A statement from the pathologists said that:

> The frequency of morbidly adherent placenta, as diagnosed by Dr Neary, was most unusual. Similarly, the clinical diagnosis of other abnormalities in the uterus, namely, weak areas in the fundus [the top portion of the uterus], was not

confirmed histologically. In fact, the Review Group were unaware of any such clinical or histological abnormality as 'weak areas in the fundus' existing in obstetric medicine.

What was Neary talking about when relaying these findings to so many mothers, such as in his chronicle of events to me? Was this, I ask, one of his spurious, self-fulfilling reasons for butchering women? I have many questions that have never been answered.

When the uterus was received by the laboratory, there would have been an accompanying laboratory form indicating the reason for the hysterectomy. If the indication outlined and the laboratory findings did not match, this should have raised alarm bells for the laboratory staff. If this had happened once, it might have been somewhat excusable, but for it to recur so frequently is unpardonable. I appreciate that there were numerous pathologists working there, so incidents of receiving a healthy uterus in the laboratory may have been spread over a number of different pathology staff. But each pathologist should have questioned their individual findings, even if they only found one such misdiagnosis. After all, this was a real woman's uterus, with a real woman's choice being usurped.

Laboratory histology reports were always returned to the postnatal ward where the patient was recovering, for inclusion in the patient's chart. Did anyone read these reports at ward level, or did they choose to turn a blind eye? If they did read them, why were no questions asked by ward staff as to why the histology findings and the indication, as written on the patient's chart by Neary did not tally, repeatedly.

The practising hospital midwives who were interviewed centred their concerns more around the young age and low parity of the affected women, rather than the act of hysterectomy itself. But why had they never before spoken publicly?

The Review Group did not find evidence that senior midwives had noted the high rate of peripartum hysterectomy in the department. Neither, as a result, did these midwives take the responsibility of enquiring from their consultant medical colleagues as to the reason for this high number. Indeed, this also applied to other medical staff, including junior doctors with access to the same patient records. This indicates inexpiable levels of patient care, and despicable treatment of mothers at one of the most vulnerable times in their lives. It further indicates that there were layers of complicity, acceptance or neglect among these medical practitioners, all of which had gone unnoticed and unheeded.

The team concluded that Dr Neary rarely consulted with any other colleague, either obstetrical or surgical, before he deemed it necessary to perform a hysterectomy.

As part of his explanation to the Review Group, Neary cited the great personal difficulty he had concerning sterilisation, which was not allowed under the hospital's code of ethics until 1997. He further stated that had he been allowed to perform tubal ligation as a means of contraception, the hysterectomy rate would have been reduced by 30 per cent. Tubal ligation is used as a permanent method of birth control. It involves shutting or tying off the fallopian tubes, thus preventing the ova, the fertilised egg, from reaching the uterus.

Herein lies the probable answer as to why he never requested assistance from other colleagues. He circumvented the code of ethics by performing hysterectomies, as this procedure was allowed, and not recording the true reason. He thought that his job would be jeopardised if he carried out a tubal ligation rather than a hysterectomy for the purpose of sterilisation.

Neary admitted that, on a number of occasions, 'sterilisation' had played a part in his decision. He also admitted that, 'The consent form might not always have indicated the prior plan.' In my opinion, this shows how, in a premeditated fashion, he fabricated the reason for surgery on the consent form. Whether this was with the patient's prior knowledge and consent is unknown, and subject to doubt. Many patients stated that they were unaware of the procedure that was carried out until much later.

Neary presented evidence which demonstrated that eight of the hysterectomies had been performed for the purpose of sterilisation. He used as an example a scarred uterus from a patient who had undergone repeated previous caesarean sections.

I cannot help wondering if *I* was that case, having had four previous caesarean sections, before Neary removed my uterus during the fifth. It gives me an insight into how 'T.A.H.' (total abdominal hysterectomy) appeared on my consent form – *after* I had signed it.

It seems to me that this covert means of sterilisation continued unquestioned. I wonder if the patients knew what was being done to them at the time of surgery. Were they fed the same rhetoric of it being a 'life-saving' operation? I certainly did not know what Neary's real plan was. Here was another clear violation, a clear invasion of the person. I cannot get inside the head of a person who continues to live a lie through such unlawful and twisted behaviour.

Consultants employed at the Lourdes Hospital had to sign contracts agreeing to abide by the Catholic ethos, as it was, traditionally, a Catholic hospital. These were the contractual terms under which they were employed. These contracts were under the ultimate control of the local bishop: the Archbishop of Armagh, and Primate of all Ireland. The ethical standards were largely concerned with the control of women's bodies: no abortion, no sterilisation, no support for artificial contraception.

I can comprehend this doctrine somewhat, as the hospital was run by the Medical Missionaries of Mary Sisters, who were, understandably, abiding by the teaching of the Catholic Church. If Neary felt that he could not work within that framework, then why did he not have the moral fibre to leave the Lourdes Hospital, where he seemed to feel so constrained, and seek employment elsewhere, where more liberal attitudes applied? His departure would have saved many women from years of anguish.

The group ascertained that because Neary was the obstetric consultant present most often in the hospital, his peripartum caesarean hysterectomy rate should, as a consequence, have been lower rather than higher. Proper antenatal and intranatal assessment would have been red-flag indicators, or signs of possible problems early on during the pregnancy and then labour, thus reducing such draconian outcomes.

Amazingly, the anaesthetists interviewed were of the opinion that all the hysterectomies performed by Neary were necessary. While I accept that they were anaesthetists and did not directly perform the surgery, they must have observed that the 'incessant bleeding' he repeatedly referred to was not taking place. They were, after all, the people responsible for checking the vital signs of the patient. Vital-sign indicators of the patient's blood pressure and pulse rate would show up as markedly declining, if a haemorrhage was occurring. They should have kept him informed that there was no cause for alarm as the patient was still stable, thus giving time to arrest the bleeding by alternative means. I would have thought that they had a moral responsibility to speak up if they noticed behaviour as serious as this, even in a single incident. One wonders if they ever even questioned Neary off the record, or expressed any disquiet.

There was no auditing of the maternity unit after Neary became team leader, and perinatal meetings or clinico-pathological conferences were not regular. The frequency of hysterectomies was just one of those things accepted by all without question.

The Review Group concluded that there were conflicting opinions about Neary's attitude to staff and patients. While some of the interviewees felt he was careful and conscientious, others, including some junior doctors, found his attitude difficult. This was supported by several examples where he was harsh or rude towards patients, and instances in which he could turn a happy event into a tense and nervous birth. His communication with management was decidedly poor. The group heard some allegations in relation to intimidation, but received no proof.

★

I experienced, in 1995, how he could turn a happy event into a tense and nervous birth. He terrified and terrorised me. Having known the man both from working with him and from being his patient, I would suggest he had both a complex personality and a personality complex.

The psychologist Carl Jung defined a 'complex personality' as 'a person with a fixation around a set of ideas'. Jung says, about personality complexes, that some people develop a set of emotionally charged ideas that reside in their subconscious. Such complexes often function as subsets to the dominant personality, and influence a person's behaviour. These complexes can be negative or positive, but are more often associated with negative behaviour. For instance, a superiority complex might influence a person to express behaviours that seem conceited.

I experienced Neary to be pleasant and polite towards many patients, but he could hurl insults at them in an instant if they asked questions he did not wish to answer, or, he felt that his authority was being undermined. You did things 'his way or no way'. He could be very witty when you were working with him in theatre, but also offensive and downright rude to staff about patients. He often made obscene references to the patient's weight, especially if they were female and overweight. Of course the patient was usually under general anaesthetic and oblivious to this. Most staff members referred to him as 'Sneery Neary', as he had a unique jocular laugh. I observed him to be heavy-handed in his surgical procedures.

Neary's use of a vertical abdominal incision as opposed to a 'bikini line' incision was perceived as out-of-date. Using this method, there is an increased risk of post-operative hernias and post-operative pain. It is also cosmetically less appealing. However, the Review Group felt that this should not be interpreted as 'bad practice'.

Whilst there were concerns about the perception that inappropriate advice had been given to patients and their families to justify perinatal hysterectomies, the Review Group were unable to comment, since they did not interview *any* patients or their families. Who made this decision, and for what reasons, has never been revealed. The review seemed like a futile exercise without this segment of information from the people involved. While his clinical insertions in the patient notes were suggestive of surgical difficulties and heroic measures, the group did not feel these were justified by the patients' post-operative states of health or levels of blood loss. His colourful insertions included:

- 'A very difficult operation.'
- 'Lucky to get away with it.'
- 'One of the most difficult problems I have dealt with.'
- 'Uncontrollable and massive bleeding.'
- 'I spent most of the night in theatre.'
- 'The most difficult obstetrical case I have ever seen.'

They found no evidence of any inaccuracies in clinical note-taking and recording – with one exception. One person interviewed stated that, in one case, as the three eminent obstetricians who initially investigated Neary concluded that his note-taking was reliable, how could they – or any other obstetrician – make a satisfactory judgement from simply reading what he had written in the charts?

The intense clinical involvement of Neary has not afforded him much opportunity for any other activities. There was no evidence that he had the opportunity to take study leave, and he has had little time to attend postgraduate meetings . . . Dr Neary has been working very hard for many years.

They recommended, on this basis, that he be permitted to return to work.

In all disciplines of medicine, especially holistic medicine, it is mandatory to engage in continuous professional development. Not having time is a poor excuse. Being too busy is an even more urgent indicator, in my view, of the necessity of continuing education in new or different practices. How can one otherwise deliver the best care with the most up-to-date medicine and procedures available?

Apart from the remarkably lax recommendations concerning Neary, another striking aspect of the Review Group's report was the reference to another obstetrician at the Lourdes Hospital, whom they found to have a hysterectomy rate ten times higher than the norm. Incomprehensibly, they did not comment on this, refer this information to the Irish Medical Council for further investigation or make any recommendations about this doctor's future practice. Surely somebody should have taken up on this revelation.

The above is only the synopsis of what I have learned of their findings from the report issued. From the outset, the report seemed to me seomwhat spurious and questionable. I find it flawed, since the central figures – the affected patients – were never interviewed. No justification for this was forthcoming. Surely the patients should have had the right to have their voices heard in this investigation. I would have thought that, if you really want the truth, you interview *all* of the people concerned before you make your final summation.

Despite their conclusion that many of the surgeries were unnecessary, they unbelievably suggested that Neary be allowed to return to work. Why?

A consequence of all these reports on Neary and into the maternity practices at the Lourdes Hospital, which follow on from his exoneration by eminent consultants, must be the unnecessary fear struck into the hearts of pregnant women, or those intending to become parents. It would not be unreasonable for parents to put all obstetricians into the same box, and, in turn, regard them all with the same sense of doubt, even though this may be largely unfounded. These reports have done irreparable damage to trust in the obstetric and general medical field.

Recommendations were made for the North-Eastern Health Board by the Review Group: that there be adequate auditing and regular weekly meetings, formalised teaching programmes for undergraduates and postgraduates, and changes to the code of ethics on sterilisation. The point that incenses most people was that they praised Dr Neary as hard-working and readily available within the hospital.

Despite finding that *half* of the caesarean hysterectomies he had performed were unnecessary, they recommended that Neary be permitted to return to work, subject to six months of postgraduate training. This is odd and frightening. It was still their view that many cases were unnecessary, and others doubtful. And yet, after Neary had left such a legacy of misery, it was the recommendation of the Review Group that he return to work.

They recommended that, for a year, a colleague should be consulted by Neary prior to him performing a hysterectomy, except in the case of an unpredictable emergency. With the majority of his cases being deemed 'emergencies', I believe this stricture was meaningless, and the probability of him including a colleague was slim and could be easily bypassed.

Were they so short of consultants that his expertise was vital to obstetric practice in the hospital?

Investigation 4: The Irish Medical Council

In the interim, the Irish Medical Council, the regulatory body for doctors, had received numerous patient complaints, and ten complaints of unwarranted hysterectomies from the public. These complaints dated from 1986 to 1990. The Irish Medical Council has a statutory role in protecting the public by promoting the highest professional standards amongst doctors practicing in the Republic of Ireland. So now began a fourth investigation into Dr Neary's behaviour.

The complaints and files sent to Dr Maresh were considered by the Medical Council. On 14 July 2003, the Medical Council's fitness-to-practise committee proved, beyond reasonable doubt, that Dr Neary was guilty of professional misconduct, and determined that his name be erased from the general register of medical practitioners. The order was confirmed by the president of the High Court, Mr Justice Joseph Finnegan, on 2 September 2003.

Neary's was said by the council to be the worst case of medical misconduct to have ever occurred in Ireland. In most cases examined and proved as unnecessary, the anaesthesia records indicated that there was no cause for concern at the time of Neary's decision to proceed in performing a hysterectomy. Even though blood was cross-matched and available, most of the patients were not transfused before that decision was made.

Neary reported to many of the general practitioners that their patient had suffered very severe bleeding, was lucky to have survived, and that the hysterectomy was a life-saving procedure. One unnamed Drogheda GP crossed swords with him over an unfounded diagnosis, and subsequently stopped referring mothers to him because of his suspicions.

The original 'three wise men', as they were dubbed by the media, were subsequently sanctioned for professional misconduct by the Medical Council. They were considered to have been negligent in a fitness-to-practice inquiry. Their misconduct was related to clearing Dr Neary, in their review, of any wrongdoing. In addition to the embarrassment of having the finding of misconduct registered on their records, they were handed the mildest of punishments, and did not face either further disciplinary action or censure. They were deemed, though, to have made a very serious error of judgement by issuing their exonerative report, recommending that this man be allowed to return to work without restrictions.

They are allowed to continue practising as obstetricans and gynaecologists. Would you trust any of these men with your perinatal or obstetric care?

★

Does it not seem extraordinary that no criminal proceedings could be – or were – brought against Neary, on foot of all of this destructive behaviour? Was there a case of collusion, collegiality, misogyny or downright carelessness? Did the medical profession, in their vindication of Neary, close ranks to protect one of their own? I am still seeking answers to these questions. No real thought was spared for the victims of this man. The reality is that, while I try to piece my broken life together after an unnecessary ordeal, he continues to walk free.

I am not and will never be totally free, and neither will many other affected women. A surgically removed uterus can never be replaced. As a patient, I felt treacherously betrayed both by what Neary did personally to me, and by the negligent acceptance demonstrated by other staff. This corrupt negligence extended into the investigations which took place subsequently, when the women involved were not given their say.

I feel unsafe, as a woman, because of the perilous actions presided over by the medical profession in conducting these inquiries. It occurs to me that this violation against women is an accepted norm in this country, which we have experienced time and again over centuries.

As a mother, I feel sickened. When a woman finds herself pregnant, she is the only person who can give birth. We are defenceless against those professionals, many of whom may be unsound people in their behaviour, who are charged with assisting with our care and safe delivery. One cannot help wondering how widespread this level of medical negligence is. Has the exposure that followed all these inquiries really stopped these practises? I do not believe so.

These obstetricians later gave evidence in the Harding Clark Inquiry. In her inquiry report, Judge Clark described these men as 'established, eminent and practising consultant colleagues, attached to the major teaching hospitals in Dublin'.

While details of their initial testimony were not published, she stated that they had serious regrets for taking part in Neary's exoneration report. They issued a collective statement, part of which said how 'bitterly disappointed' they were at the findings, which were 'fundamentally wrong'. But it appears that the 'regret' only came after the independent consultant, Dr Maresh, had disputed their findings and they had misconduct charges logged on their records.

There are so many unanswered questions about which I would dearly like to interrogate these men. Was their regret based on Neary being caught up in malpractice? Or was their sorrow based on being caught themselves, I wonder? What was the 'prevailing situation' that they referred to? Was their report based solely on an 'old boys' club' mentality? Why were we so 'fortunate' as to have an obstetrician who denied so many women the chance to have further – or in some cases any – children? On what basis did they make that assumption, and where was the good fortune in being terrified to death? What was their clinical judgement based on? Does that cosy cartel which operated then still exist in Ireland, in other areas of medical care? Did the patients whose files were examined matter to anybody? Should they not have been the first to be informed of the findings, and kept abreast of the ongoing investigations? Imagine, an organisation investigating itself.

It is my firm conclusion that power corrupts, and absolute

power corrupts absolutely. Neary wielded the unquestioned, absolute power which was bestowed upon him, with military precision and domination. There is absolute power which only God possesses, and He is incorruptible. In my opinion, Neary thought himself incorruptible. He played at being God.

Chapter 10
The Government's Reaction

Investigation 5: The Lourdes Hospital Inquiry

Vast amounts of public finances had already been spent on ascertaining what happened. I wondered, though, as we headed into a fifth inquiry, why it had taken so many. To date, most reports had concurred on several points. So was there much more information that another investigation could uncover? What was missing from the previous investigations and subsequent reports?

Consequent to the Medical Council's investigation uncovering a number of alarming facts, in 2003, the Lourdes Hospital Inquiry was established. Following preparations and appointments to the board, the inquiry was established on 6 April 2004 by the then Minister for Health and Children, Micheál Martin. It would be conducted by Judge Maureen Harding Clark, but the terms of reference were later agreed by Minister Mary Harney.

The terms of reference included:

- Examine Lourdes Hospital's peripartum hysterectomy rate from 1992 to 1998.

- Ascertain the system of recording such hysterectomies at the hospital, and ascertain whether all expected records were extant and, if not, what had happened to them.

- Inquire as to whether Dr Neary's practice was commented on or acted upon by colleague consultants or other medical, nursing or management staff within the hospital.

- Inquire whether any review or consultation with others took place following such surgeries being performed.

- Examine what mode of clinical reporting took place, and what actions applied thereafter.

- Examine the adoption of new practices and protocols arising from the publication of the previous reports.

- Advise the Minister for Health whether it was necessary to add other protocols or systems.

- Inform the Minister of any staff dissent, poor or total non-cooperation with the inquiry from within the hospital, should this arise.

Witnesses were initially reluctant to present for interview, but this improved, with almost 100 percent of witnesses invited eventually attending. The inquiry subsequently received widespread cooperation. Three hundred, twenty interviews were conducted, with 280 witnesses, including former patients, midwives, sisters of the Medical Missionaries of Mary, retired and practising obstetricians, IT specialists, statisticians, nurse managers and matrons. This was the first time that evidence directly from former patients was included in an investigation.

One colleague consultant of Neary's was willing to attend the inquiry, another was undergoing surgery and another had an illness in the family. Neary indicated his unwillingness to attend, but was prepared to answer questions by letter. Interestingly, Neary was not compelled to attend.

I received a letter asking me to attend the tribunal of inquiry at Bow Street in Dublin on 23 February 2005. I had previously never had reason to appear before a judge, and I did not know what format the proceedings would take. Was I going to a courthouse? Would there be a presiding judge and jury? Would the public be there when I was giving my evidence and being questioned? As I had not been given any insight into the protocol of proceedings, I was so full of trepidation that I again began to feel really panicky. It was almost as if I was guilty of what this man had done – as if I was on trial for some crime I had committed.

I took the bus to Dublin, for the interview, on a wintry February day. Upon arriving at Bow Street I was visibly shaking. I immediately realised that it was not a formal courthouse, but this did little to comfort me. Though it was a bitterly cold day with heavy snowfall, I was sweating and terrified as I walked up those stairs. Judge Clark thought my sweating and tremulous condition was due to the inclement weather conditions, and suggested that I take a few moments to compose myself and get warm, but in reality I was once more in a state of extreme panic. Once again, I had broken down.

Judge Clark and her assistant were pleasant and professional towards me. She invited me to sit across from them at a large desk covered in files and legal papers. She listened carefully to my evidence and my story, sometimes shaking her head in dismay. She frequently asked if I needed a moment to compose myself. She sympathised and empathised with my plight, reiterating that in her view, *all* of the women who had suffered at Neary's hands should be compensated for this most horrific ordeal. She pointed out, though, that she could only work within the terms of reference set out for her by Minister Harney. She also pointed out that this only included those who had verification from other obstetricians of the hysterectomy operation being unnecessary. I felt like she was gently preparing me for failure.

Basically, the psychological repercussions were not being taken into account. The interview lasted over an hour, but I became visibly upset towards the end. I was aware that, once again, I was being dismissed, this time by Judge Clark on behalf of the Minister for Health. Of course, it was not her fault, as she was working within the remit which she had been assigned.

As I left that building after the interview and walked down Bow Street, I felt downtrodden. In my heart, I knew that I was being excluded from any of the compensation that I was entitled to, that my situation did not matter to anybody and, as such, that it went unrecognised. My life felt worthless. I just kept walking aimlessly, crying profusely, knowing that I didn't matter. At one point I was startled by an elderly gentleman who gripped my arm, asking, 'Are you all right, love?' He had compassionately observed my distressed state.

I scarcely noticed the heavy snowfall except to periodically clear the snow from my glasses. I had already wasted so many years of my life, and my family's life, on something that I had been subjected to but was not responsible for. All the pain and suffering I had endured, much of which was continuing, was irrelevant to others who were supposed to care. I had spent any available money my family had trying every conceivable therapy and treatment to improve my health. Once again, that perilous monster was whispering in my right ear, telling me that my family would be better off without me. I was, after all, the cause of their young lives being turned upside down into dreadful turbulence. I had spent the money that should have been saved for their future education. And now I knew in my heart, from Judge Clark's body language, that I did not matter, under the guidelines that she had been given.

That bus journey home was spent trying to hide the unstoppable tears from other passengers. Once again, the dam had burst. I felt this was my last chance to be heard, and I had assumed that I did not have any further avenues to explore.

My suspicions were confirmed in a letter from the Redress Board on behalf of Justice Harding Clark, dated 31 October 2007. An excerpt from Judge Clark's letter reads as follows:

As you are no doubt aware, it is a condition precedent to inclusion for assessment of redress that an opinion be furnished from an obstetrician or gynaecologist, who has examined the applicant's medical notes, that the operation was medically unwarranted in all circumstances. For those reasons I regret to inform you that the circumstances of your application did not give rise to an award.

During the initial announcement of the establishment of this inquiry, Minister Mary Harney stood up in Dáil Éireann and proclaimed that: 'Every woman injured by Dr Neary must and will be compensated.' This is not what happened. To me, it seems that Ministers Harney and Martin's knowledge or understanding of 'injury' was narrow, unenquiring, misinformed and merely relating to the physical. Or, was it simply another political rhetorical device, to pretend to the public that this scandal was being addressed by the government? The inquiry consequently merely looked at the physical outcome of the patient.

Talk is cheap, and words can be as hollow as an empty canister when there is no follow-through. Why was 'every woman injured' by Dr Neary not compensated or included in the expensive tribunal's findings? I have no idea how much these inquiries cost, but I expect it ran to several million euro. The real winners were the legal people, while many of the victims were ignored, without compensation even for the medical expenses they had personally incurred. In truth, many women were left penniless as a result of Neary's actions, and the ensuing actions of others.

Terms of redress for compensation included which pregnancy the surgery applied to, and the age of the mother at the time. They did not address the psychological damage inflicted by what one media article dubbed 'Drogheda's butcher boy', unless *all* criteria were met. Why was this?

★

As human beings, we are holistic complexes comprised of four levels: physical, mental, emotional and spiritual. When injury takes place, it takes place on all four levels.

Physically, I had been injured not only by the act of a very questionable and unnecessary hysterectomy, but also by the making of a hole in my bladder. This hole was enlarged for no apparent reason aside from Neary's own pleasure in suturing. There have been serious and lasting problems left in the wake of this. For me, this was a clear case of misadventure and neglect.

Mentally, Dr Neary instilled fear beyond belief, culminating what I took to be a clear death threat towards me and my as yet unborn infant.

We are well aware that what happens to the mother at any stage during her pregnancy affects the baby in utero, due to the proximity of their spinal columns. This includes any shock the mother receives prior to the birth, including trauma, as it crosses the placental barrier to the unborn infant. Yet medically there was never any treatment offered to me or my daughter to help deal with the shock. This abiding fear is far more deeply ingrained in my psyche than any physical scars, of which there are many.

Emotionally, I had also been seriously injured. As documented in my notes, I requested counselling. Little heed was given to this request, by nursing staff or Dr Neary, despite Dr Neary's knowledge of my previous experience of postnatal depression, following the emergency delivery of my second baby. I wonder if he had some fear that his own actions would be disclosed if he offered or consented to further referral? This also happened to my request for allergy testing for anaesthetic components, which was scoffed at by Neary in 1986. Surely, giving me a prescription for Prozac was assuming a diagnosis, even though he was not a psychiatrist, rather than coupling with or opting for onward referral for counselling. Perhaps he was afraid that a counsellor would probe his actions. In truth, I feel emotionally raped by this man.

Spiritually, I was traumatised and questioning the love of God, or even if God could exist. I felt so abandoned that I wondered if this was something I deserved.

I was excluded from compensation on the grounds that I could not get an obstetrician to vouch that my surgery was unnecessary. They also stated that I had agreed in advance that the procedure was necessary. How could this have been recorded, as I *had not* agreed to such a procedure? 'T.A.H.' (total abdominal hysterectomy) was written on my consent form *after* I had signed it, and without my knowledge. This led any reviewing consultants to believe that I had consented to the hysterectomy by Neary prior to surgery. They probably thought that I was dishonest, and seeking financial compensation. This is totally untrue and does not come into my moral remit. It is what I know in my heart that matters.

In addition to this, part of my notes, those kept in Dr Neary's private rooms, went missing and remain unrecovered. While missing files was one of the criteria for compensation, in my case, this was not taken into consideration. There was a clear case of attempting to minimise damage, and make the number of cases involved look as few as possible, or make the number of mothers injured appear as small as possible.

Many files from the hospital's records department mysteriously disappeared. The chairman of the Medical Board condemned the theft of the files, suggesting that the issue was a matter for the Gardaí and office of the Director of Public Prosecutions. Whether such an investigation took place I do not know, but, to my knowledge, there were never any charges made for this offence. No public proclamation on this was ever made. Judge Harding Clark was constrained by the parameters set out by Minister for Health, Mary Harney and the hospital notes of patients, as presented to her.

Judge Clark's findings were made public by the Tánaiste and Minister for Health Mary Harney, in February 2006. This was also the day of my mother's death, at the age of seventy-two. Mam was my strongest supporter through it all, my greatest advocate, who constantly stood by me and encouraged me to do whatever I had to in my attempt to seek justice and regain my health. That fight for justice still goes on in her memory. She was very conscious of any media attention given to the case, and would immediately call to check on my wellbeing if she saw Neary or anything related to him on the news. She knew the effect that his appearance on television or in the print media had on me – I would be very unwell for days. She was deeply disturbed by what had happened to me on that fateful day in July 1995. She worried constantly as she observed the change in my demeanour and behaviour. So many times she said: 'I am heartbroken by what has happened to my only daughter. I feel so helpless watching you fade away and I can do nothing to stop it. This will kill me.'

Mam developed an aggressively rapid thyroid cancer in January 2006 and was dead in three weeks, despite being given a prognosis of nine months. The thyroid is the organ of communication and has a special affinity to the mother-child relationship. I believe that emotional hopelessness leads to cancer, and that the depth of her grief for me accelerated her illness and death. This led to further guilt and remorse on my part, as I felt that I was destroying lives, including the life of my own mother. Had I not been sick,

I wondered whether this fate would have befallen my mam. The void that has been left in my life after her death is immeasurable.

Snapshot of the of Judge Clark Inquiry findings

Judge Harding Clark issued a comprehensive report on the inquiry findings. She concluded that it uncovered a story of unquestioning submission to authority within the Lourdes Hospital. There was a real sense of toeing the line and minding your job within the hospital. The small but busy hospital seemed to obey rules unique to itself, unaccountable to what would today be regarded as objective medical standards. An excerpt from Justice Clark's report stated that:

> Neary was neither an evil man nor a bad doctor, but a doctor who at critical points during his training was inadequately supervised. It is the story of a doctor with a deep fault line and a misplaced sense of confidence in his own ability.

Judge Clark did not elaborate on her 'deep fault line' theory. 'Few complained or questioned', she said. It is evident from this how convincing he was.

The inquiry found the number of peripartum hysterectomies performed by Neary 'truly shocking'. Between 1974 and 1998, a total of 188 peripartum hysterectomies were performed at the Lourdes Hospital. Of this figure, 129 cases were performed by Neary. Once again, one wonders why nobody said 'Stop.'

Neary's patients were generally younger than the rest of the maternity unit clients. Judge Clark said that most of these mothers also had fewer children. She concluded that 'Neary's antenatal clinic included a higher proportion of problem pregnancies, with a higher ratio of repeat caesarean sections than the other consultants'. I can only wonder who diagnosed these 'problem pregnancies'.

I would also question who had performed the previous caesarean sections: was it he was in fact responsible for some of these? There are many young mothers attending maternity units all over Ireland; young motherhood is not peculiar to Drogheda.

Another conclusion reached was that none of the obstetricians working with Neary were aware of his tendency to resort to early hysterectomy. Because ward rounds were shared amongst all three consultants, I find it hard to believe that, when covering Dr Neary's off-duty hours, the other obstetricians did not raise an eyebrow at the high number of hysterectomies they saw performed. Anaesthetists retrospectively felt that he may have been too quick to resort to hysterectomy, but did not imagine that they would be consulted on this matter. Nor does it seem that they questioned or attempted to intervene, even to suggest that he seek a second opinion.

'Pathologists assumed that some hysterectomies were sterilisations, but said that they were unaware of the cumulative numbers carried out in the unit.' Could this be true? They too must have been aware of the code of ethics within the hospital, and have chosen to ignore it. Each case they examined should have been scrutinised, if they felt unhappy.

Some junior doctors expressed gratitude to Neary for assisting them in emergencies. Other junior doctors, however, described unhappy experiences with the consultant. The lack of meetings,

teaching and discussion was a notable cause of such disgruntle-
ment. In fairness to the junior doctors, they all needed his reference for their curricula vitae. This, and their relative inexperience,
probably stopped them from speaking out about what they
witnessed. This included, in my opinion, the reigstrar, who
assisted my delivery in 1995. He may, I suppose, could have been
minding his position and watching his future reference.

Between 1978 and 1979, the matron had expressed concern
to one of the senior consultant obstetricians about the high
number of hysterectomies carried out by Neary. Her concerns
were said to have gone unheeded. She was told not to worry;
Dr Neary was afraid of causing a hemorrhage. She felt that this
senior consultant was indicating to her that she should back
off. She then tried speaking to the other senior consultant, who
responded, by gesturing, that she should not persist. She was
afraid to speak out, as she believed that Neary had been
reviewed by the Medical Council, and that his practice had
been found to be acceptable. I wonder could she have not at
least checked this out further, as this would be the duty of a
matron? Who or what was she frightened of? Was this an indicator of the collegiality amongst the consultants in the unit?
Did it further indicate that they did not want to know what
Neary was doing, and refute the statement that they were
unaware of the number of hysterectomies he performed?

A temporary midwifery tutor also expressed concerns, but
did not contact any outside clinician, the medical director, the
pathologist or the senior obstetrician. Was this due to her 'temporary position', or her keeping an eye on her career? One of
the 'whistleblower midwives' came to work at the hospital in

September 1997. She was taken aback by some of the practices she observed there. She, along with another midwife, made her concerns known to the North-Eastern Health Board during that fateful meeting in October 1998. That was the first real action, throughout all levels of staff, taken to protect the mothers attending this facility.

The Royal College of Obstetricians and Gynaecologists inspected the maternity unit in 1987 and 1992, and deemed it to be suitable for training obstetric registrars and for undergraduate training. Strangely, no return visit was planned, following recommendations made in 1992 to ensure that they were implemented. On neither occasion were the recommendations suggested fully implemented.

An Bord Altranais carried out periodic midwifery school assessments for accreditation purposes. In 1980 they advised that women should be offered a full choice of contraceptive methods, with midwives to be fully trained on these methods. Nothing happened and no such training or implementation occurred.

In considering the report prepared, with Neary's input, by the three consultants, Judge Clark concluded that their report was prepared to enable Neary to continue working. They had serious regret for their part, but admitted that they were motivated by compassion and collegiality. In simple English, there was an attempted cover-up.

Regarding the missing files of Neary's patients, the inquiry found that an unidentified person(s) with knowledge of where the records were stored was responsible for a deliberate and systematic removal of key historical records, master cards and patient charts, which were now unaccounted for. Additionally, three alterations to the maternity theatre register were detected; these complains appear to have been made by the same person after complaints were made against Neary. Again, I suspect that my chart was among those that were tampered with. Justice Clark concluded: 'Someone with a misplaced sense of loyalty to Dr Neary or the unit is probably responsible. The missing files seriously hampered the inquiry by the absence of critical records.' Secondary records and the information given by patients had to be relied on in such cases in the Justice Clark Inquiry.

In May 1997 the North-Eastern Health Board formally took ownership over the Lourdes Hospital from the Medical Missionaries of Mary. This was the first hospital founded by Mother Mary Martin. The sisters were very dedicated, and ran the hospital in an orderly, austere way, and with excellent fiscal-management practices.

I had completed both my general and midwifery nurse training there, under the auspices of the sisters, and I would reiterate that most of the time they were firm but fair with students. Of course, like all institutions, there were some strange occurrences. For example, I was once on night-duty in the general hospital. I had put an egg on to boil for a patient's breakfast, but had gone to pray with a patient who was dying. During this time the patient died and, of course, I forgot about the egg. When the assistant matron came to do her early-morning rounds, she observed the egg in the now boiled-dry saucepan. I was summoned to walk down the six flights of stairs, holding the egg on a spoon, to tell the matron that I had wasted an egg.

They certainly operated a very different hospital from that

which exists today at Lourdes or, indeed, most other hospitals. What is the accepted norm today – long waiting times, endless rows of patients on trolleys in public areas – did not occur during their reign. At least, that was my experience. And yet, it does not seem to me that our population has grown so much, or that the finance given to the hospital is now much less. One cannot help but wonder what has gone wrong since the sisters left the Lourdes Hospital, and with other hospitals. In my opinion, it is not more money the sector needs, but better administration of what is available.

When the Medical Missionaries of Mary sisters (MMMs, as I will refer to them in future) were interviewed by the Judge Harding Clark Inquiry team, it was put to them that a uterus would have previously been removed because of its friable condition or for the purpose of sterilisation. In response, they requested that the following statement be included in the records of the inquiry: 'The MMMs would like it specifically stated in the report that they were not given any specific information in regard to the fact that this occurred, though it appears to be accepted by the inquiry.'

This statement is very questionable, since many of the wards had MMM sisters in charge for most of this time span. In the period between 1945 and 1997, only two matrons had served, whom I feel sure had regular meetings with the MMMs on what was happening on the ground. Many staff had been there for most of their lives – for many it had been their first and only place of employment. The hospital was probably the largest employer in town. One has to question whether this lent itself to a collegial loyalty, or to turning a blind eye in an attempt to keep a job.

The inquiry team formed a strong suspicion that a number of planned hysterectomies were done for sterilisation purposes. Sterilisation was not permitted within the Catholic ethos of the hospital. However, 'indirect sterilisation' was allowed where the primary purpose was to protect the mother's health by means of hysterectomy.

'For every adverse comment the inquiry heard about Neary, they heard one in his favour, with several patients convinced that he had saved their lives', the inquiry reports said. Perhaps he did, or was this part of how he convinced patients to accept what he was doing? He certainly had me convinced for quite some time. For many mothers, they were not informed that they had undergone a hysterectomy until much later in their postnatal period. Those who challenged him for carrying out the procedure found that Neary's attitude became defensive and unfriendly. Perhaps this was part of his personal conviction of being right, or his reaction to being caught out.

Judge Clark concluded that major changes had taken place in the maternity unit in the wake of the Neary revelations and the reports that ensued. The incidence of peripartum hysterectomy had fallen precipitously, she said, and now accorded with national standards, and midwives had updated their skills and attended management courses.

The inquiry found that 'the Lourdes Hospital had been caught in a time warp without badness or cover-up. Hard-working, decent staff had unwittingly enabled bad practice when support and safety systems were not in place.' Is this excusable when the lives of so many women were destroyed? If these people were in any other employment, I feel sure that they would be sacked and possibly face criminal charges for negligence.

'Dr Neary's air of competence and confidence in the theatre and other areas of obstetrics and gynaecology concealed his defensive practices and masked appreciation of his fear of haemorrhage from colleagues,' Judge Clark concluded. This affirms my opinion of him having either a complex personality or a personality complex, or, more likely, a little of both.

★

I suppose that you are on the point of saying, 'My dearest Kathleen, where were you when all these inquiries were going on, and what was happening for you?'

The fact that I have taken some time to include what was happening in the external world after the whistleblowers came forward was to brief you on the Health Board's pursuit of the facts of what happened in the interim.

Truth is, all through this time I continued to contain my suffering in panicked, fearful silence. I was attempting to exercise non-judgemental compassion towards the circumstances and people who had turned me into a shattered wreck. I believed that this is what God wanted me to do. My deep feelings of hurt have meant that I cannot.

All the while, I was (poorly) attempting to uphold some level of normality at home and get my children educated and maintain our home life. But it seemed as if I had been valiantly struggling for an eternity. So many times, my strength became so depleted, my purpose felt extinguished. My hope seemed like an abandoned ship in the midst of my despair.

All the while I was working and spending my earnings on therapies.

Chapter 11
The Redress Scheme

Following the findings and recommendations of the Judge Harding Clark Lourdes Hospital Inquiry in January 2006, the government proposed to provide compensation for patients affected by Dr Neary. The scheme's objective was to compensate those who underwent unnecessary obstetric hysterectomies and bilateral oophorectomies (removal of both ovaries) as certified by an external examiner. The government approved this scheme on 18 April 2007.

Those eligible to apply for compensation under this scheme included those who had experienced:

1. An unplanned obstetric hysterectomy, which in the opinion of a consultant obstetrician was medically unwarranted.

2. Along with an oobstetric hysterectomy, an unplanned bilateral oophorectomy, or the removal of single remaining ovary where, in the opinion of a consultant, this was unwarranted.

3. An unplanned obstetric hysterectomy where the woman's relevant hospital records were unobtainable.

4. In association with recent pregnancy, a dilation and curretage (D&C) or evacuation of retained products

of conception (ERPC) or examination under anaesthetic followed by an unplanned hysterectomy which in the opinion of a reviewing consultant was medically unwarranted.

5. Bilateral removal of both ovaries or the single remaining ovary while the patient who was still under forty years of age and which was subsequently medically deemed as unwarranted.

Women who were not eligible to apply included:

1. Any late applications.

2. Women who had already received compensation through court or other settlement of claim.

3. Any woman who had been advised by an outside consultant reviewing her records that such procedure was appropriate at the time and in all the circumstances.

4. Any woman who agreed in advance with Dr Neary to have any of the operations on an elective basis.

The ex gratia payment was calculated by:

1. Age at date of unwarranted obstetric hysterectomy.

2. Number of children at date of unwarranted hysterectomy who survived at least six weeks.

3. Maternal age on date of unwarranted bilateral oophorectomy or of obstetric hysterectomy.

4. Age at date of unwarranted bilateral oophorectomy.

Dependent on the criteria set out, recipients were awarded, in some cases, up to €180,000.

> The ex gratia offer of redress so calculated is intended to take into account all injury, psychological trauma, loss and damage suffered by the applicant arising from the listed unwarranted operations.

But, as I well know, this is not what happened in reality. Where applicable, there was also accommodation made for legal costs. Once again, the legal profession were the winners.

Despite part of my records being missing, despite 'T.A.H.' being added *after* I signed the consent form, I was denied any compensation or reimbursement of the costs I incurred. This included exclusion on the grounds of trauma caused, as outlined and agreed in the terms of reference set out.

Given my experiences, I find this deeply unjust and inhumane. I have spent seemingly endless amounts of money in a quest to get well, because of unnecessary injury caused to me by Dr Neary and others. And yet, this was never considered, assessed or addressed. Where is the justice in this? Was the Hippocratic oath of 'first do no harm' ever considered?

Chapter 12
Discovering That My Case Was Under Scrutiny

It was a routine day at work in 1999 when Arlene, my daughter, who is also my secretary and clinic manager, requested that I take a personal telephone call. This was unusual, as telephone calls are not taken by therapists during treatment sessions except in a real emergency. But she relayed that this call was from my GP. It was unusual that she should call me, and I immediately thought that something must be seriously amiss. She began by asking if I was having any ongoing problems or concerns after my hysterectomy surgery. We had a brief chat as to how things had been since I had been in hospital, before she gently broke the news to me that she had been contacted by the North-Eastern Health Board, enquiring if I was well or had had any problems. My understanding of her telephone call was that she had been asked if I needed help since mine was one of the hysterectomies now under investigation.

I was stunned. This was the first that I knew of any investigation into my hospital records. I had been through a psychiatric incarceration, and only now were they asking if I needed help. Had they known all along that I was unwell, I wondered? I never did receive help from the Health Board, with the exception of them paying Professor John Bonnar's consultation fees (which I will explain later).

Why could the Health Board not have contacted or notified me directly, I angrily thought. I wrote to the chief medical officer in August 1999 outlining my situation, and requesting an explanation and answers for what was happening.

I sent the letter to the North-Eastern Health Board, and asked if my hospital records were included amongst the charts being examined and, if so, why I had not been previously notified rather than my doctor. I subsequently received a letter dated 9 September 1999 from Jim Reilly, acting senior executive officer. It read:

I refer to your recent letter addressed to the chief medical officer and which has been passed to me. I would be obliged if you would contact Ms Lambe, patient liaison officer at Our Lady of Lourdes Hospital.

And that was the sum total of the reply I received from Mr Reilly. I read and reread the brief content of this letter in amazement. My initial thought was how contemptible the brevity of his reply was about such a serious and personal matter. I found this succinct response lacking in compassion.

At that point, I was finding existing on a daily basis difficult, often impossible, so to have to begin contacting the patient liaison officer, who I did not even know, seemed like a hill too high to climb right then, such was my level of fatigue, distress and illness. I did nothing immediately, because I was still too unwell, both physically and mentally, and barely operating. I felt like a number.

In October 1999 I was admitted to the Lourdes Hospital, having collapsed, and suffering chest pain and dyspnoea (difficulty breathing). This had now become a regular occurrence for me, with the least extra ripple of stress in my life triggering symptoms. While in the coronary care unit, I heard the patient liasion officer's name being called over the public address system. I nervously decided to request a meeting with her to discuss what was going on. Ms Lambe was pleasant and compassionate. She was one of the first people with any humanity and compassion I had encountered in all of my ordeal. She was so willing to listen, and made me feel as if I was important. She made me feel like she had all the time in the world for me – because I mattered. This was not a scenario I had been used to while I had been seeking answers.

We had a frank discussion of the entire ordeal and its repercussions. I explained my confusion to her, and she fully understood because, as she said, she had listened to similar stories from many other women. I challenged her on the claims that Neary had 'saved my life'. But with the progression of time I now know that I was still in disbelief, still hoping that I had not been so badly betrayed – otherwise I would have definitely spoken out sooner. I did not want to believe that any human being could be so evil.

Ms Lambe expertly explained how the inquiry had come about, culminating in her statement: 'Your story is a replica of what I have been hearing from other mothers. Kathleen, this is not your fault. Believe me this is not your fault, you have done nothing wrong.' She proffered further private advice, and advised that I speak with my GP again for further referral and assistance, which I did immediately following my discharge from hospital. I felt for the first time that someone was listening to me and empathising with my situation.

★

On this occasion, the GP suggested that I see a gynaecologist to ascertain if my ovaries had been removed, in an attempt to explain my ongoing ill health. My hospital chart stated that my ovaries had been left, but who could I believe now? Why was I so unwell?

I was referred to a doctor in Cavan, whom I saw and paid for as a private patient in November 1999. I found her approach brutish and heavy-handed, and did not feel that compassion was her greatest attribute. She performed an ultrasound scan and a trans-vaginal scan. She said that this was the only sure way of determining whether or not the ovaries had been removed. As she walked back towards her desk she unambiguously stated: 'Well, Dr Neary must have put your ovaries in his pocket, as you don't have them, and they do not appear to have reached the laboratory.'

In a weird sort of way I was relieved to get a diagnosis. I hoped that it could somehow explain – even justify – the myriad health problems I had been experiencing since July 1995. The doctor assured me that she would send a report to my GP. I telephoned her on numerous occasions, leaving messages with her secretary – but still no response was forthcoming. This was followed on two further occasions by sending registered letters requesting the report, but still no reply. I then contacted my solicitor, who both telephoned and wrote to her office, but this did not produce a response either. I was, and remain, mystified by her inaction. I did not receive this report until the summer of 2015 (see Appendix A). Is it not obvious that there was a cosy collegiality here, a mentality of not letting your colleague down? This doctor was next appointed as Dr Neary's successor at the Lourdes Hospital.

Why did she refuse to furnish this report for so long? Either she made a correct diagnosis, or she did not. Until this episode I did not realise that a doctor could refuse to furnish a report on their patient, even to that person's GP.

★

Each expensive obstetric review consultation I attended did little more than dent my confidence in the medical profession, increase my negativity and put me deeper into financial debt. At this point I had spent several thousands of pounds, and many more euro, in seeking a solution to my poor health. This was money which I could ill afford. It was as if the medical fraternity were closing ranks against me in an attempt to protect Neary and his colleagues. I felt as if they were hoping that I would go away.

For me, and for most human beings, fear of death is the greatest fear imaginable. Since the entire drama of threatening me and my baby with impending death was unnecessary and irresponsible, it is my solemn belief that, for his actions, there is a clear case against Neary. In my opinion, what he did was premeditated.

I wrote to Ms Harney many times, and telephoned her office repeatedly. Each time I called I was unfailingly told by her secretary that she was in the Dáil chambers, that she was considering my case and that they would call me back. But of course, this was all idle talk as they never did contact me. Her office personnel were just fobbing me off. In fact, I often felt like they were laughing at me. I must have made several hundred calls to her office, all in vain. I can't help but ask if any of my messages ever even reached her. Every human being is entitled to an answer, even if it is in the negative.

Subsequently, I wrote to all politicians of all parties in the Dáil. I have lots of paperwork to prove they were 'looking into my case', but again, this was idle rhetoric, with no further follow-up. They constantly make declarations of what they would recommend and do, but, from my experience, this is just idle chatter for public consumption. Not a single TD followed through on their promise 'to look into my case'. Each member obviously has their eye on their own seat, but cares little about the issues of the Irish constituent. With the latest change in government, I renewed my search for justice, as healing is hampered without justice. I have sent correspondence to An Taoiseach Enda Kenny, Dr James Reilly and other politicians, but still await concrete action. Despite the strong advocacy, on my behalf, of one young Fine Gael TD, my quest continues unanswered. He has taken a very keen interest in my case on a personal level, partly perhaps because he is a solicitor by profession. He recognises the injustice done to me.

In February 2000, I spoke to my solicitor, also a family friend, who agreed to write on my behalf to Ms Lambe, the patient liaison officer, as suggested by Dr Reilly. Ms Lambe acted swiftly, and immediately passed this letter on to the deputy chief executive officer of the North-Eastern Health Board, who responded with this astonishing reply to my solicitor: 'I refer to your letter dated 22 February 2000, addressed to Ms Lambe, patient liaison officer, Our Lady of Lourdes Hospital, and which has been passed to me for attention.' His letter continued:

In October 1998, the North-Eastern Health Board became aware of concerns regarding the clinical practices of a consultant obstetrician gynaecologist at Our Lady of Lourdes Hospital, Drogheda. The North-Eastern Health Board requested the Institute of Obstetricians and Gynaecologists in Ireland to assist in a process of reviewing the clinical practices of the consultant concerned. The chairman Dr Harold Lamki set up a review under the chairmanship of Professor Graham Harley.

The Board referred a number of patients' records to the Review Group including your client's records. The Review Group then undertook an assessment on an effectively anonymous basis. The board has no way of knowing whether or in what manner your client's records were considered by the Review Group.

In anticipation of queries similar to those raised in your letter, the board asked the members of the Review Group to identify the particular patient records they examined, and the conclusions reached in respect to individual patients, but the Review Group declined to do so.

The board has an added difficulty in that, on the conclusion of its report the Review Group immediately disbanded and therefore does not any longer exist and, as such, is not available to the board to deal with queries of this nature. We therefore regret that we cannot assist you with your query.

Can anyone comprehend receiving such correspondence from a health board steeped in this inquiry, especially after they had been in contact with my GP to ascertain whether I needed help? It was as if they were operating on separate lines. What was the purpose of contacting my GP? Were they hoping she would quietly reply to their query without letting me know? But the overriding issue for me was the fact that my health had been destroyed, yet nobody seemed to care. It seemed as if the health board personnel were operating on several different levels. I wished that they could spend a day in my life at that time: they would surely run scared. There seemed to be no place for real human beings in their world. It was as if there was a prevailing mentality of covering it up, minimising the reality and getting off the daily news headlines as quickly as possible. I found this letter deeply disturbing as, once again, I felt that I was just an insignificant, anonymous number. If the content of the deputy chief executive's letter was entirely true, then it meant that nobody was identified by the report – that it was non-specific in its findings regarding any individual concerned. What was the point of such a costly exercise?

I felt that the Irish government were willing to allow taxpayers' money to fund inordinate fees for investigators who would either not report their findings specifically, or for whom the criteria set out were so spurious that it did not explicitly request this information in the terms of reference. After all, this was not a normal routine spot check, but rather an investigation into one of the biggest scandals Ireland has ever seen. If a breach of confidentiality in releasing the identities of the patients had been the worry, then surely the Department of Health could simply have been kept out of the public domain. A lot of money could have been saved in the classification of those patients whose surgery was deemed 'unnecessary' by identifying the victims the first time round. Additionally, it would have saved time – and harrowing sadness – for the many women who had to pursue long and tedious means in seeking the truth. I find it cynical that investigators could be paid handsome fees while many of have spent our own money in a quest for wellness after externally inflicted ill health. We, the women who were affected, were reduced to being ID numbers rather than human beings who had been mutilated.

Could the government not have passed emergency legislation compelling the Review Group to identify those affected, and disclose this information to the Minister for Health, with the purpose of compensation in the name of justice? Was this an indication of the government's acknowledgment? Was it due to there being no watchful eye looking out for the citizens?

Chapter 13
The Court Case That Never Reached Court

My search for potential solutions to my health problems continued incessantly. Then, in 2002, I found psychiatrist Dr Michael Corry. Michael practised a combined holistic and allopathic medicine approach, as opposed to a solely medical model. Our paths had crossed when I was a general nursing student, as he was at that time interning in obstetrics and gynaecology. I consulted with him at Clane Hospital but, as money was scarce, I could not attend for appointments as often as I needed or would have liked to. Dr Corry strongly suggested I be admitted to Clane Hospital for deep sedation, but I declined as I could not face another hospital incarceration. His diagnosis was immediate. Below is an excerpt from his report:

> The events of 10 July 1995 had an enormous impact on the life of Kathleen Ward. She developed a serious post-traumatic stress disorder, which remains unresolved. This was by any standards a terrifying experience. In contrast to her pre-morbid personality, she is but a shadow of her former self. The revelations that started to emerge in 1999 regarding Dr Neary's possible malpractices were an enormous source of distress to her. For her there has been no

escape from the facts surrounding Dr Neary's malpractice. Her source of pain is ubiquitous, and prevents psychological and emotional healing. This is what makes her situation so tragic and her prognosis so bleak. She remains a broken, trapped individual whose well-being is spiralling out of control . . . I have rarely come across such a tortured individual with such a poor prognosis.

Michael had worked with Dr Neary as an obstetric intern, with the intention of becoming a consultant obstetrician and gynaecologist. He described Neary as a misogynist, who completely put him off following his intended career path. He told me that he had seen Neary conduct procedures that were both outdated and dangerous, and had no place in modern medical practice.

He related to me, on more than one occasion, that the only chance I had of recovery was to face Neary in court. He felt that this could help break the cycle in which I was trapped. It was my version of locked-in syndrome.

Court scared me so much that I kept putting off his suggestion. I did not feel like I had the mental strength to face it. In truth, I also didn't have the mental stamina to cope with seeing Neary in person, which would no doubt happen at some stage during the court case.

However, in 2004, I decided to take Dr Corry's advice and face Neary in court – my health was on a roller coaster heading nowhere. If there was a possibility that eyeballing Neary in court would bring me some closure and healing, then I had to do this, irrespective of how difficult it might be. *Could things get any worse than they already are?* I asked myself.

I kept insisting to my legal team that I wanted to serve proceedings on the grounds of post-traumatic stress as a result of his negligence.

There was – and is – no doubt in my mind that Dr Neary lied to me, betrayed me and violated me, causing hurt beyond belief, and that what he did was common assault. Even if – which I sincerely doubt – the procedure he executed was entirely necessary, it is not the role of any doctor to terrify the patient (which I felt was for his own personal satisfaction), whether for secondary gain or because of personal shortcomings.

There was no abnormal blood loss recorded, my vital signs were stable and neither I nor my baby were dying, so surely the need to reiterate imminent death was reckless behaviour. This is the behaviour that caused the PTSD in the first place, so I assumed that this was reasonable grounds on which to base my court case. My biggest challenge was post-traumatic stress, and I wanted to challenge him for causing me such harm by his conduct. My legal team advised me that such a court challenge against a member of the medical profession had never before taken place in Ireland.

Advice was coming at me from all sides, most of which kept insisting that another, better grounds for the court case was to base it on the unnecessary hysterectomy. I had to find an obstetric consultant to vouch for that claim. I knew that this would be difficult due to my altered hospital chart. To this day I feel that unlawful hysterectomy was the premise on which to pursue the case.

I was referred, in March 2001, to a consultant at a Dublin clinic, for medico-legal opinion. This involved substantial cost.

I asked the North-Eastern Health Board for assistance, and they agreed to pay. However, I found that meeting both frustrating and infuriating. The consultant read through my notes, looked at my healed but well-scarred abdominal incision, and asked a few brief questions on my current state of health.

As I was replying to his questions, his telephone rang and he took the call. This, of itself, I found most unprofessional. He had a very jovial conversation, which included whether or not he should wear a tuxedo to an event he was invited to. I sat there gobsmacked: he was claiming a substantial fee from the North-Eastern Health Board and using part of such sensitive consultation time to have a light-hearted, private conversation. His actions displayed a massive disrespect for his client and a total lack of empathy towards my situation or any shred of professional care. This person was a regular television speaker on the Neary subject, presumably earning fees for doing so. My own experience as an owner of a clinic made me question whether he was simply conducting the appointment for money, rather than out of concern for the patient.

I became weepy as a result of his personal manner, and the fact that he took the telephone call. I once again had the experience that I was not being listened to by a doctor. Though briefly acknowledging my anxiety and depression since the hysterectomy, he stated that the operation was not the cause of my problems, and that the surgery was, of course, necessary. At that point he had lost me, and I felt a deep disrespect in his approach. This doctor was an obstetrician and professor in obstetrics, but not a psychiatrist. It was as if, at any cost, he was determined to vindicate Neary and the wider medical profession. I felt misunderstood, as though he was trivialising the pain, hurt and misery I was going through, with no understanding and no desire to gain any.

As I was leaving his consulting room, his final farewell was that my hysterectomy was necessary, and that what I needed now was good psychiatric care for depression. He told me to give up the 'alternative medicine nonsense', and return to midwifery. 'We are very short of midwives, you know.' And for this advice, he was paid.

I left his office utterly in pieces. I felt so humiliated by his callous disregard for my situation. I felt like he had placed himself in the position of adjudicator, earning a handsome fee in the process. In retrospect, I feel like he was attempting to put me off any further investigation of Neary's conduct. What gave him the right to dish out opinions on what profession I choose to follow? I have practised holistic medicine for thirty years; I wonder how much knowledge he has of the profession or what it really consists of. Many detractors of holistic medicine base their claims on hearsay and ignorance, rather than the much-needed assistance we give our clients, and the many who consult us as a result of disillusionment with the medical profession.

Proceedings were lodged in the High Court but, as I could not find a gynaecologist to state that my hysterectomy had been unnecessary, they seemed doomed from the outset. I will never understand why I was fobbed off. I suspect that the addition of 'T.A.H.' influenced their rejection. I will probably never get an answer.

My solicitor, realising that I did not have a medical report which stated that the surgical procedure was unnecessary, was becoming increasingly uneasy about achieving a positive outcome: he felt that I would be fighting the system. I had by now made contact with the group Patient Focus in Drogheda, as I had heard them referenced in relation to the Neary case in the media. I was invited to attend a meeting in Drogheda, accompanied by my solicitor. I expressed my fears and concerns to Sheila O'Connor, national coordinator of the group, about the financial implications for me if I lost the case. She encouraged me to press on and go to court.

Patient Focus was established as an advocacy group in 1999, providing a point of contact and support to patients who have been damaged by the Irish health care system. They claim to have a unique insight into and expertise on the Irish health care system. Among other goals, their list of aims includes:

- Ensuring the preservation and enhancement of patient rights in all health care settings.

- Assisting people to try to resolve difficulties as early as possible.

- Providing primary loyalty to patients with ready access to their organisation by telephone, fax or email to the patient or their family.

While they state that theirs is not a membership organisation, but rather a registered charity, it is unclear where their funding comes from.

Initially, Dr Neary's legal team attempted to block me from taking my case, on the grounds that it was statute-barred from the courts due to the length of time since my surgery. This, however, was overturned. In June 2004, at the request of my solicitor, the solicitors for Neary and the North-Eastern Health Board consented to a High Court adjournment for two weeks, and no longer. My solicitor requested this as I was once more unwell. Each time it came close to the court date, I went into an emotional meltdown, and had to seek adjournment on those grounds. I feel that the solicitors figured that I would not be emotionally strong enough to face court, and that by applying further pressure they would scare me into withdrawal.

My legal team told me that if I lost the case, court costs could run to about €300,000. I was scared that I could lose my home, as there was no other way that those costs could be financed. Considering all of that advice, I was left with no option but to withdraw my case and not go to court. To this day, I regret that decision.

Leaders of Patient Focus were infuriated by my decision to withdraw, and subsequently quietly cut all ties with me. I was never notified of another Patient Focus meeting nor of any future developments in the compensation scheme.

But sharing the glory or commiseration on the courthouse steps would not keep a roof over my family's heads. Prior to my withdrawal from the court case, the national coordinator of Patient Focus, Sheila O'Connor, had given me her home telephone number, and advised me to call her any time I needed assistance. On one occasion after my withdrawal, another redress scheme was announced for those excluded in the first redress. I heard this on the RTÉ 6:00 news, and called Shelia shortly afterwards to enquire if I could possibly be included in this scheme. She curtly told me to stop calling her at home; if I had a question I was to call the office instead.

This, for me, brought their aims into question. I felt very let down. If it was their intention to assist people who had been harmed physically, emotionally and psychologically by health professionals in Ireland, then surely cutting off a patient in need was a breach of their own rules. I felt, from this experience, that they were as adversarial as the system I was fighting. Their attitude raised a lot of questions for me in relation to their 'unique insight' into the Irish health care system.

These incidents might seem like insignificant everyday setbacks to most folk. I may even be coming across as a whinger. The truth is, though, that I am yelling now because nobody listened when I spoke nicely. When you are already finding doors closing against you, feeling fragile and ignored, then this series of events could serve as another tipping point to end it all.

The damage brought to bear on Irish women by Neary, and those involved in the mishandling of the case and the misman-agement of evidence, should not just be forgotten. Too often we see murky scandals being covered up and minimised. Take the symphysiotomy redress situation, which I will explain in chapter sixteen. There is an attempt being made, in my opinion, to silence these women by offering them a choice: that they either take the compensation offered and waive their legal rights, or get nothing. This surely cannot be called justice. I will not be silenced. I will expose this scandal whenever the opportunity arises.

Now that the court case was off the agenda, I went through the highs and lows of another emotional roller-coaster. On the one hand I was glad that I did not have to attend court, but on the other there was a sense of finality. I felt like I was on the M1 of life, with no slip-roads to get off and seek help.

Chapter 14
How I Have Been Affected by Dr Neary's Actions

To realise that one decision made by another individual changed the direction of my life so drastically reminded me never to take for granted the life path that I was called to journey on. I did not physically die on 10 July 1995, but my spirit died, along with a large part of my soul. In the years since then I have every day felt like my life was over. Any time I saw Dr Neary on television or in the press, I became emotionally distraught, as if he had come right into my living room, as if I was being attacked all over again. Friends told me that it would get easier, but in fact, for a long time, it seemed to get harder, which was very confusing. Human nature leads people to forget over time what they are going through, and this made it more difficult to cope, as everyone wondered why I was so lifeless and why I retained such vivid memories of the events. Unwittingly, I spent so much time emotionally hiding – hiding from the public, from clients, from friends and family.

Since that fateful day, my health changed irreversibly. For years I did not feel well. I mastered the art of putting on a mask in public, while inside I felt like shattered glass. I experienced so many negative emotions, including depression, loneliness and emptiness. I felt completely alone in the world, with a feeling of unreality, a sense of being in a vacuum and of being 'locked in'. It was as if my inner being had gone into freeze mode: an internal state of paralysis which could not be unlocked. I no longer felt free.

I was so indescribably tired that it was difficult to work. It was the sort of tiredness I hear clients speak about who suffer myalgic encephalitis (ME or post-viral syndrome).

I would be in bed as early as 7 PM, or at the latest, by 9 PM, so as to be somewhat functional the next day. This was very unsettling to family life as I was in bed before the children, which disrupted their childhood. Before 10 July 1995 I would read to the children at night for hours, but now I was either asleep or just fretfully lying in bed, often crying, even before they lay down. No amount of sleep was recuperative or refreshing. I would swing between total insomnia for several nights, feeling too fearful and terrified to sleep, to sleeping so deeply that I could scarcely wake up in the morning. Dreams were recurrent, especially the nightmare of seeing myself above my dead body. Of course, I now realise that sleep not being recuperative is a symptom of extreme stress and anxiety, even depression. Normally, when we sleep our brain and our body calm right down to *shen*, or inner peace. But while my body was exhausted, my mind was like a greyhound in full flight.

Intense stress allows the body to drift off to sleep, but the brain keeps going like a racehorse, unable to reach a level of inner stillness, leaving both mind and body in an ongoing state of chronic fatigue. Eventually, we enter the general adaptation stage: 'GAS' as we call it medically. This is where the body accepts, on some level, the abnormal stress in an attempt to survive, but the whole body cannot keep going in this mode over the long term if this abnormal level of stress continues. I should have been off work, but I could not afford this. I felt trapped in a no-win situation.

Life no longer felt enjoyable. Instead, it was replaced with frequent, almost constant illness, irritability, anger and frustration. I was full of trepidation and guilt. I worried about everything – everything was a crisis. This state was all new to me, and I could not cope because I did not know how to. I rarely got out socially, partly due to lack of money but also due to fatigue, fear and lack of interest. This was unhelpful and added to my isolation, as friends became fewer. I did not go the cinema for fifteen years. In the past we had enjoyed going dancing and to hear country bands; now we barely remembered what a band sounded like, or when we had last stepped onto a dancefloor. Peter might make plans for us to go out, but then I would feel tired and 'down'. I would go to bed rather than get dressed up for our night out. My television viewing now only consisted of news bulletins, checking for any updates on Neary. In brief, our lives were dictated by my emotional state, so making plans to socialise seemed impossible. This was the new spiral that we, as a family, were stuck in.

Close friends who knew me pre-1995 would say that I had a total personality change. I became very withdrawn, introverted and uninterested, always wanting to be alone. Fun and laughter were no longer part of life for me: this was part of my 'hiding'. I felt constantly sad and bereft, like I had died but was still here, as if I had been raped or sexually abused. I felt lost in the fog of the imperfect journey of life. Nobody chooses illness, but you are rarely given a choice when it hits you. The greatest friend of depression is solitude, and that was what I was living.

Daily panic attacks left me with a fear of fear. I experienced chest pain and indescribable panic followed by fainting on numerous occasions, and often ended up in the coronary care unit. An example was in 2002, when I awoke at 1 AM with a blistering headache and was admitted to hospital as an emergency. So intense was the headache that, on reaching the hospital, doctors initially thought I either had a sub-arachnoid (brain) haemorrhage or meningitis. The ultimate diagnosis was, as always, extreme stress and panic. If clients unwittingly mentioned Neary, I would freeze and have to leave the room to do breathing techniques. Every day was a silent hell. I felt destroyed inside.

My husband agonised in silence for all those years. He was terrified by this new reality which hit our family. After all, I had simply gone into hospital to have our baby and now I was an emotional cripple. Our life and our relationship had changed irreparably. We were like tense strangers living together. He has never really spoken about the effect it has had on him, or sought help for his own trauma, or the total upheaval in his life.

My family life with my children suffered badly. I no longer felt like a proper mother or wife. In some way, I was always sick, tired and irritable. I could not relax, lighten up, sing or have fun any more. I endured but rarely enjoyed life.

I often identified with a statement which Annie Maguire of the Birmingham Six said of her wrongful imprisonment: 'I looked through the prison bars at my children, helpless to reach, touch, advise or enjoy them. I watched them grow but only from a distance.' That summed me up in one statement. I have felt imprisoned for the past nineteen years, and my sentence started on 10 July 1995. It is a prison without walls, without chains and with no chance of remission. Above all, there was no release date. That indelible mark has been imprinted on my brain like a tattoo.

My ongoing emotional condition was also a large influence on my decision to withdraw from antenatal teaching. The Lourdes Hospital maternity unit was within my catchment area, so Neary's name would inevitably be mentioned by parents-in-waiting. These women had no idea of my experience with him. Their comments unknowingly connected to that part of my life, and they invariably triggered extreme unease and panic in me.

Despite having been a very successful antenatal teacher for many years, I had to stop teaching as I no longer had confidence in the Lourdes Hospital. I no longer had confidence in me. I no longer had confidence at all. I felt that I needed to warn people of the potential risks attached to that institution. But of course, I realised that this would be reckless advice as the delivery of these mothers' babies would be fairly close by the time they reached the antenatal class, and I certainly did not want to instil unnecessary fear in these women – that was not my role. So the best option for me was to stop teaching.

On one hand it was a decision that I made with relief, but on the other hand – and in truth – I had lost my nerve. I felt heartbroken; I loved teaching. I also needed the income more than ever to support my family, but I could not live and work with how I felt. Once again, I had to listen to my conscience.

Fast-forward to 2012, when I decided I was ready to teach again. Going through the greatest recession in history, the survival of many businesses was deeply uncertain. I wanted to tick all boxes and batten down the hatches to ensure the survival of our clinic, so I was exploring every avenue possible to extend what we could offer. I also felt that I had a lot of experience and knowledge to impart. But this return was not as easy as I had expected.

Despite doing a refresher course at University College Hospital, Cork, I found the main local hospitals, Our Lady of Lourdes in Drogheda and Cavan General Hospital obstinate in their approach. Both hospitals were attempting to keep all classes within their own units, whether that suited the mothers or not. Not all working mothers can get time off for such events during the day, and I was offering evening, full-day and weekend classes to suit. In the Lourdes Hospital they even refused to display a poster advertising my classes: one midwife told me that she faced being reprimanded if she was seen to promote classes outside of their unit. 'Why?' I asked. But she failed to give me a reason other than to say that it was hospital policy. Have they now closed ranks entirely?

At Cavan Hospital a poster was reluctantly accepted, but placed outside the staff canteen, well out of view of mothers attending for their antenatal visits. In fact, one midwife I approached there asked me, 'Do you feel that mothers really need to attend classes?' Other antenatal teachers I have been in touch with have encountered similar attitudes from both units, so it was nothing personal.

My view on antenatal classes is very clear. To do any job in life one has to do a certain amount of training, from the most menial task to professional work. Yet, to be a parent, it seems one just has to get pregnant, and deliver a baby, and one is suddenly expected to be an expert. As a parent we wear many hats: we are mother and father, nurse and doctor, psychologist, referee, teacher, taxi, cook and a whole lot of other things. Does that not require training? In the past, many new parents had the benefit of advice and assistance from their own parents, grandparents and other extended family. Demographic change has altered that dynamic for many, so, many new parents must learn on their own. Antenatal classes are a necessary beginning in education, but should also be the beginning of another point of contact if help or advice is required at any time during parenting.

When I teach antenatal classes I include much more than labour preparation: I aim to prepare new parents for what lies ahead. I cannot comprehend why a midwife would ask if antenatal classes are necessary. The biggest fear mothers and fathers have going into labour is fear of the unknown. If they are prepared for what lies ahead they are less afraid. Surely this only makes the work of the midwife a little easier, when that mother comes into hospital prepared. Security and strong bonding with a child from birth to age seven is critical. I worried about not being present for a lot of that period in my children's lives, especially my youngest daughter's. My bonding with this baby was badly fractured, as I was neither physically nor mentally present for many of her early years. I rarely took photographs of her, did the fun things I had enjoyed with my older children at that age or took her away on day trips, as I had an inordinate fear of driving. This time can neither be relived nor revisited. Naturally, she became and still is very close to her dad; he was everything to her during those early years. I remember her once asking me, 'Mammy, when can I spend time with you?' This ripped my heart apart, yet I felt incapable of addressing the issue. It was reliving Annie Maguire's experience. So many times I felt that the children would be better off if I was no longer here. What always stopped me was fear.

I feel sure every parent has moments of feeling like they are a bad parent, but on top of this, I have had fears that my children would remember me as a wicked, dysfunctional mother; I hope that my fears are unfounded. Childhood lasts a lifetime, and I worry that their memories may be so scarred that they may become traumatised, dysfunctional adults.

Thankfully, so far they are hard-working, well-rounded young adults, never bringing a moment's trouble to our home. I am immensely proud of all of them and their respective achievements. I am so grateful for their support and resilience; without their love and encouragement I would not have survived. My 'baby' sat her Leaving Certificate this year and excelled, and has now left home for college. This was, as expected, a very poignant time, as she is still the special baby, the miracle.

Since the death of Dr Michael Corry, I had been in a search of a therapist with a similar holistic vision and ideals. In 2012 I discovered Dr Harry Barry, who was then a practicing GP and cognitive behavioural therapist working in Drogheda. Dr Barry has written many well-known publications on mental-health issues. When I read his 'Flagging' series I instantly recognised that he 'got it' – that he was inside people's heads in his understanding. He believed in dealing with the causative factors rather than merely the symptoms, or worse still, just numbing the reality with medication. I found his sessions very helpful and always came away with the feeling that someone was finally 'hearing' me. That was the major turning point in my recovery. So committed is Dr Barry to assisting people with emotional issues that he is now practising cognitive behaviour therapy, as well as lecturing and writing.

★

I am thankfully now, by and large, in a much better place emotionally. Nevertheless, I still experience many black days. I feel like I could carry the hurt and injustices to my grave if I let myself. Life will keep bringing us the same test over and over again until we pass it. My new motto is 'Start by doing what is necessary, then what is possible.' Gradually I find that I am doing the impossible – like writing this book. In the words of my grandmother: 'Man forgives and remembers. God forgives and forgets.'

Chapter 15
Not Being Defined by 10 July 1995

Over the past nineteen years there were many times when I felt as if my life had been split in two, especially in the years just after 10 July 1995. Each half felt fragmented and splintered. My very being was operating on separate planes most of the time: survival plane or business plane. On a physical and emotional level, I was in robotic survival mode, moving up and down the panic scale, my moods like a kite in a hurricane. It is like being in a rapid lift which takes you from the ground floor to the sixtieth in ten seconds.

The moment somebody mentioned anything that offered a view of Dr Neary that was at variance with my own, or a manner or attitude that I disliked, the shutters came down and I switched off – into panic mode. This would catapult me right back into hiding, once again cocooned in my own little world. Hiding from what, even I do not know, but it was that time during my progress through the various phases of the human condition when I could not cope with life.

After enduring many years of fruitless and wearying struggle to attain the unattainable, I had to look towards an ultimate, distant goal. I once described it as 'like trying to build a house using a teaspoon'. In a sense, I had come round the corner and was heading slowly into the light. What was current in my life was not working, so I had to look for alternatives. For so long it was as if there was a voice inside my head, asking if I would ever live again before I actually died. Most of the time there were no concrete answers forthcoming, simply because there were none. But equally, I realised that life was too short to live the same day twice. Of course, my improvement did not just come with a sudden awakening. Rather it was as a gradual result of all the help I have received. It is still interspersed with some bad days.

Neary had almost succeeded in extinguishing the last of the old Kathleen, but only almost. There is an old Kerry saying that truly applies to me: 'It's not the size of the dog in the fight, rather the size of the fight in the dog.'

Beneath it all, I was determined not to spend the rest of my life on the garbage heap. For too long I had shunned my other self, the caring mother and wife, holistic medicine worker and nurse and midwife, work which I had trained so hard and so long for. It was, after all, my passion, as I have devoted my life to the well-being of others.

I was the only one still hurting, not Michael Neary, so with each new dawn I prayed for the strength to get joy back into my life. Prayer, without a doubt, helped save me and, for that, I thank God. Throughout, I heeded the advice my dad gave me all those years before: 'Kathleen, never forget your prayers.' Even though there have been many times when I cried, 'My God, my God, why have you forsaken me?' I kept prayer as the central focus of my life. I believed that in darkness, faith is the light. I prayed to have eyes that would let me see the best, a heart that would allow me to forgive the worst and a soul that never lost faith. In my heart I knew that only God could turn a mess into a message, a test into a testimony, a trial into a triumph, a victim into a victory. I realised that I was trying to control everything around my emotional state, but that, as a consequence, I was enjoying nothing and feeling out of control. My new motto is: 'So what if I panic – let it flow and it will pass as it has done in the past. Panic will not kill me.' I realised that it was time to let go, and let God take over.

So began my daily routine of even stronger prayer: praying hardest when it was hardest to pray. I still like to rise at 6 AM and offer prayer and thanksgiving for an hour. This is a great time, as the house is normally quiet, and there is real personal time for God and me to talk, and the most satisfying spiritual breakfast I can enjoy: real prayer. I hoped that if I could accept what is, let go of what was and have faith in what will be, that ultimately I would 'pass the test', and God would step up to the mark in helping me move forward into the next phase. God does not sit and have a chat, but He has gifted me with a great sixth sense, among many other gifts. He has sent many blessings into my life. And He did step up to the mark.

Because of our financial circumstances I was left with no choice but to continue working at the clinic. I did this on a gradual basis, within a few months following my release from hospital in 1996. This was not an easy transition. I felt how hard and fretful it was to begin to acknowledge that lost part of me. What will people think of me? Will they shun me now that I have been ill? Am I capable of really devoting my life to 'alternative medicine nonsense', as indicated by the consultant at the Dublin clinic? My confidence and self-esteem were gravely dented. I was not lost, but did not know where I was going. I needed the financial income to support my family, and I also needed to safeguard my sanity by having less time to think of myself. Moreover, I knew that I had a lot to offer to others to help them improve their lives. If anything positive came from my personal experiences, it was a deep empathy and compassion for the suffering of others. In life, you can buy anything except experience, and I had the knowledge and the experience to serve the sick. Sincerity only bears fruit when it is nourished by wisdom. So, once again, I let go, and let God take over. After all, there are no coincidences in life, only 'God-incidences', and even therapists are allowed to get sick sometimes.

Appearances are deceptive. Outwardly, few would have suspected that anything was wrong in my life, especially my clients, who were unaware that I was ill, and even fewer still were aware of what had happened to me. Many would comment on how I had it all, how lucky I was to never need a doctor. When I was at work I became completely immersed in my clients: I switched into a different gear. From life's experience, it is my conjecture that, when we suffer anxiety, stress or depression in our lives, we develop an 'ism'. We create a crutch to help us cope, or as a means of putting off facing the inevitable. In psychological terms it is called a displacement activity. People often develop drug dependency, eating disorders, alcoholism, or workaholism. I believe I developed the latter, workaholism. I suppose I had a bit of that in me from my childhood. My parents had a loose theory, that 'when you could walk you could work'. Idleness was not accepted at home. I worked more and more, longer and longer hours, in an effort to build up my business: this was part of my 'ism', I suppose.

We must have the only house in Ireland with three garages built in our lifetime, yet none remaining. When my mother-in-law came to live with us all those years ago, we converted our first garage into a granny flat and built another garage onto that extension. After her death, we converted the granny flat and garage number two into clinic space, and built number three. I wanted to separate the house from the business to allow for family privacy, since my family was getting bigger. At this point I had brought in another vega-testing therapist like myself, as I could not cope with the numbers seeking to attend the clinic.

Vega-testing checks all organs in the body. It measures energy, allergies, pH, infections, geopathic stress, emotional stress, depression and much more besides. It gives us a holistic picture of where the client is 'at' on all four levels, thereby guiding us to the best possible individual treatment. I just did not have time or energy to see the volume of clients who were now seeking appointments. I was and am also a practising reflexologist, naturopath, herbalist and antenatal teacher.

My colleague additionally practises acupuncture and Chinese medicine, and remains working with me all these years later. I was approached by a chiropractor asking if he could join our team, followed by a physical therapist, so we needed additional space: garage number three had to be converted.

Nine years ago we moved to a purpose-built clinic, still at my home, but completely separate to my private house, as we were continuing to expand our range of therapies. In addition to the other therapies, I have now added an osteopath who has many additional qualifications. I also have a cranio-sacral therapist who specialises in cranial fluid dynamics, which deals with stress. She also practises cranial osteopathy.

I continued trying to build up my clientele, most of which I did by word of mouth. Our clinic was novel, as there were few holistic clinics of our size in Ireland at that time. Part of what makes us different is that we listen deeply to our clients' stories and assess their needs on all four holistic levels.

I want to be a success, to be the best in the business along with my carefully selected team, and I do not accept failure lightly. Thank God we are achieving fantastic results for our clients, by and large. Of course, we do not always cure everybody. If there was one therapy that cured everybody, we would surely be practising that. Constructive criticism is always welcome as a means of ongoing learning and improving what we do. But we sometimes find that what criticism there is comes from people who want a quick fix, which doesn't exist. My therapists say I have eyes on the soles of my feet, as I constantly have my finger on the pulse of what is happening within our walls.

Arlene went on to college at the National University of Ireland in Maynooth. She studied biology and mathematics, and graduated as a secondary-school teacher. She always had an affinity for holistic medicine, and studied reflexology alongside her Maynooth studies. After teaching for some time, she realised that teaching was not for her, so when a vacancy came in the clinic office she jumped at the opportunity to join the team. She is now clinic manager and reflexologist. She is married, with two beautiful children.

When Karen left secondary school she pursued a degree in tourism and marketing at the Dublin Institute of Technology, but she decided to return to further education and become a primary-school teacher, which she loves. She too is now married.

Edel completed an arts degree at University College Dublin. Then she whizzed around the world for a year. On her return, she too pursued further education and is also a very happy primary-school teacher. She is getting married later this year.

Padraig had an avid interest in farming from a very young age. So it was no surprise that when he left school he went to Ballyhaise College to study agriculture. He later attended Dundalk Institute, where he qualified as a carpenter. He is getting married next year to his beautiful fiancée.

Kerrie has always been the artistic girl in our house. Little wonder then that she has chosen fashion and design as her career, and turns out some fabulous creations. She is in her final year at the Borders College in Galashiels, Scotland.

Caoimhe has been accepted into St Angela's College, Sligo. There she has commenced her course in home economics and religion, with the intention of teaching in the future.

All these years were like being a juggler, marrying family and business life, all while enduring emotional challenges. Now that the family were living more independently, I often prayed, *Give me a big break, Lord.* I want to emphasise that I am no 'holy Joe' – but a day without God would be meaningless. This is where God really came in, and stepped up to the mark.

Let me preface this by saying that, within the clinic, we all carry, at my express wish, a copy of the code of ethics of the medical profession. Whatever happens or is said in my clinic, stays in my clinic unless revealed by the client: there are no exceptions. In 2004 I was approached for consultation by Ryan Mellon, a noted County Tyrone footballer, who had been very ill for some time. Ryan had been doing the rounds of the medical profession, but not achieving the express health outcome he desired. Shortly after commencing treatment with me, a tragic event struck his life: his football colleague and great friend, Cormac McAnallen, died from sudden cardiac arrest. At the time it was thought he had died from a virus. This was terrifying for Ryan and his family, as indeed it was for all the team members. I was treating Ryan for a virus at the time. Ryan thankfully responded well to our regime of treatment. He got better and better until, within a very short time, he was able to return to football again.

In September 2005, Ryan proudly lined out for the Tyrone team again. They were playing Kerry in the all-Ireland football final on that great third Sunday in September. Make no mistake about it, I am inseperably attached to the green and gold of Kerry. However, on this occasion, Kerry were beaten by Tyrone, with Ryan playing no mean part in that defeat. While on one level I was disappointed for Kerry, I was (secretly) equally immensely proud of Ryan for his part in that winning team. I remember going into the bathroom and shedding a tear of pride for Ryan, and thanking God for his recovery. Having watched this talented and personable young man go from not being able to get out of bed to proudly lining out in Croke Park on all-Ireland final day, I realised that my life's gifts were worth something to others.

Amazingly, on his way to the post-match victory celebrations, Ryan telephoned me with his thanks. This is something I will never forget; it touched me deeply. In his moment of glory he remembered someone who had helped him, and I found this very honourable. This call meant more than

'Thanks' – it gave me a reason to go on, a belief that I was not a total failure, a belief that I was doing something right. I felt as if God was reminding me that, when I worked with the right premise in my heart for those I served, he was observing. Apart from some colleagues who were involved in Ryan's treatment, nobody outside of the clinic was aware that I was treating him, unless he had told them himself.

Nothing, however, could have prepared me for what lay ahead. The following Sunday afternoon I was busy sorting out the children's school uniforms for Monday morning and preparing food for the two girls going back to college. The family were doing their own thing at football, meeting friends, while the youngest two played with Barbie dolls. My second daughter burst through the front door shouting, 'Mammy, mammy!' I initially thought she was late for her bus to Dublin, so I scurried into the kitchen. She excitedly exclaimed: 'Have you seen the *Sunday Independent*? There is a full-page article about Ryan Mellon and you.' I froze. My usual sense of panic momentarily overpowered me, as I wondered *What have I done wrong?* That sense of self-doubt was never too far away. But I need not have fretted: Ryan had been interviewed by the *Sunday Independent* on his marvellous comeback. He had chosen to tell his story, and talked about how I had helped him, in this article. I was unsure how I felt. I was overcome with emotion.

Before that day was out, the phone was ringing incessantly, with people calling seeking cures. The calls came from everywhere: mostly from footballers, hurlers and golfers, but also from the general public. They came from the four corners of Ireland and beyond, seeking help with ailments. Were it possible for me to be cloned, I could have set up clinics in every county, such were the requests and invitations to do so. To this day, clients still refer to that article from all those years ago. In hindsight, I realise I missed an opportunity that could have helped my clinic grow even further. Had I had the confidence to give interviews to the media, it could have been a huge break for my career, but leftover fears from the past can so easily haunt our present moments. Perhaps it was not meant to be at that time. This newfound fame put the clinic on a different plane, as it got busier and busier, and thankfully remains so.

The years since continue to be very busy. There is scarcely an ailment that we have not been presented with. Somehow we started to treat more people with infertility problems, and had great success, for the most part. My private office is covered in photographs of those beautiful babies, whom I call 'my babies'. There is nothing more wonderful than to help a couple bring new life and joy into their world.

Continuing to explore and expand, in 2010 I brought a test to Ireland, which is for early detection of heart disease, one of Ireland's most common causes of death. I have now been appointed national coordinator with responsibility for training new consultants, so this is taking me on another tangent. Apart from this, we see and treat all types of conditions, such as back problems, chest ailments, stomach and bowel ailments – virtually all illnesses. I have even been doing a voluntary radio slot monthly with LifeFM radio on health issues, which I thoroughly enjoy.

In 2010 my clinic was shortlisted for the Small Firms Association Outstanding Small Business of the Year award. While I did not win, I was in the final ten, which was a great honour.

Following on the heels of this business recognition came my greatest and most appreciated surprise in 2012. Once again, I was working with clients when Arlene called me for 'an urgent phone call'. As I picked up the handset, I asked Arlene who was looking for me, but she pretended not to hear me and scurried past into another office. The lady said: 'Hi Kathleen, Aine Toner here. Congratulations, you are in the final twelve.' Not knowing who Aine Toner was or what the final twelve meant, I replied: 'Ah yeah, right, but I think you have the wrong person'. I was sure this was some prank call. But Aine persisted saying: 'No, no, your daughter Arlene has nominated you for *Woman's Way* Mother of the Year 2012, and you are in the final twelve. I am the editor of *Woman's Way* magazine.' I was truly speechless. I cannot remember what I muttered as Aine laughed, realising that I had no idea about this. Aine quoted an excerpt from Arlene's letter to her:

I really don't know how she keeps going or where she gets her energy from. Without her and dad we would be lost as a family and as true friends. Thousands of others would also be lost on a health basis. She has a strong work ethic and exceptional mothering skills. She has an ability to work through whatever life throws at her; life has been far from rosy for her and that makes mam a real winner in my eyes.

Aine told me there was a lot more in that letter, which moved the judges immeasurably. She told me that she needed to do an interview, and proceeded to ask me some questions. One side of my brain was answering questions, while the other half was asking myself many more. *What did she say? What else is in that letter? How will I face the final judges?* I never did find out the rest of the content of that letter that Arlene wrote.

The final gala was held in the Westin Hotel in Dublin. It was an auspicious occasion for me; I was accompanied by Peter and Arlene. There were four provincial winners, and I was crowned Ulster Mum of the Year 2012 based on Arlene's nomination. We were showered with many beautiful gifts at the event. Of all the pleasant things that have ever happened in my life, I found this the most moving and emotional, as I felt really appreciated by my family. When my name was announced, I just sat there, then burst into tears. This event taught me that I must be doing a lot right in my life, and that the fears are only within myself: only I can – and must – address them. Since family are my life's purpose, this award meant everything to me. Thank you Arlene, so much.

While life has thrown me onto many cobbled paths, I appreciate that most people are given their crosses to bear. I realise it is important to always look forward and rarely turn back. Now I see each day as a blank page in the diary of my life. The pen is in my hand, but the lines will not always be written the way I choose. Some will come from the world and the circumstances that surround me. The secret of life is in making my story as beautiful as it can be, even with the struggles I face.

Integral assets in my recovery have included:

- Following my dreams.
- Working hard.

- Being kind to all.
- Ensuring that smiles are always returned.
- Having fun.
- Not focusing on what I lack.
- Realising that other people are the true treasures in life.
- Taking daily exercise.

Certainly in the excercise department, I initially struggled. I could find twenty-six excuses not to get out and exercise, often reducing myself to tears, then giving myself that last push out of my comfort zone and just doing it. This is such an important part of recovery.

Remember, right is right, even if nobody is doing it; wrong is wrong even if everyone is doing it. Goodness will always be rewarded.

Chapter 16
Trying to Make Sense of It All

Much has been written about the events surrounding Dr Neary and what actually happened, and why nobody sounded the alarm over twenty-five years. How his actions could possibly recur so frequently without the intervention of other medical profession-als remains a mystery. What was it all about – for Dr Neary, per-sonally? Many journalists and authors have professed to have the answers, but the fact is that only Neary has the real explanations. In my opinion, the real cause will never be known; Neary will carry this secret to his eternal reward.

The year in which it was noticed that an inordinately high number of these needless hysterectomies was performed, 1996, was also, sadly, the year that his wife prematurely died. This led people to speculate that, as a result, he was either inspired by vengeance or consumed with an irrational fear of cancer. But this was scoffed at during the inquiry. After all, how could this explain all those previous years of unnecessary surgery?

Dr Neary has never explained his failure in his duty of care to his patients and has never apologised for his actions or the suffering he caused, which is criminal. He has never given a reason as to why he created these emotional minefields, which left women scarred on all levels by abuse inflicted over a twenty-five-year period. He has never acknowledged how he has ruined lives, destroyed families and the possibility of having future children, leaving couples either completely childless or with fewer children than they had wanted. Children are the jewel in the crown of life: when another chooses to destroy that gift of life, we are losing precious jewels.

The irony for me is the conflict within Neary himself. Writing in the *Irish Independent* on 4 March 2006, journalist Medb Ruane wrote:

At one place, he seems to claim that the hospital's religious ethos contributed indirectly to the high number of procedures, because practices such as sterilisation were forbidden there. In other words, he sees himself as a hero circumventing what was allowed. Elsewhere however, he ironically claims that the reason he left obstetric practice in the UK in 1974 was because he took a stand on principle and wanted a conscience clause to spare him performing sterilisations and abortions. There, if true, he was a hero for exactly the opposite reason: what a contradiction in his following years of practice. Yet, on another level he was slicing women open from the navel down and removing the very soul of their femininity, ensuring they were sterile into the future. While he insisted that he acted in the patients' best interests, his absolute certainty that he was right, is itself of major concern.

His vocal friend, Sheila Martin from Drogheda, furnished the *Irish Independent*, in March 2006, with a photocopied a letter sent to the secretary of the Department of Health in December 1993, in which Michael Neary wrote:

I have been informed by various Medical Missionaries of Mary that failure to implement their policies in this matter [the ethics code] could result in my dismissal from the unit. We have been quite prepared to abide by the rules as laid down by the Medical Missionaries of Mary.

This letter raises even more questions, as it appears that the MMMs themselves must have raised concerns about his code of conduct in regard to the hospital's code of ethics. What were the MMMs so perturbed by to have threatened his dismissal? Why would this letter have been necessary? It seems contrary to evidence given to the Harding Clark Inquiry by the MMMs, when they seemed 'surprised' by the revelations of his hysterectomy rate. I find it hard to believe that some of the Sisters would not have noticed what was happening as they were a part of the hospital workforce, with Sisters working on all wards, mostly in the role of Ward Sisters. Additionally, despite the content of Neary's letter to the Department of Health, he carried on circumventing the sterilisation ban by performing hysterectomies, according to his own admission, to the inquiry. How immoral was this practice, and how unnoticed or selectively blind were those who were supposed to be keeping a watchful eye?

This culture of acceptance seemed to extend beyond the MMMs and the Lourdes Hospital. Subsequent governments, including the government at the time of the inquiry, also seemed afraid of challenging hospital procedures and shortcomings. This was evident in the Madden Report on organ retention, and then subsequently in their fear of challenging or prosecuting Neary.

The public inquiry was only instituted following national public outcry. Ms Harney said, on publication of the Harding Clark report, that the question of compensation 'did not arise at this time'. What was she thinking, and where was her care for the women affected? Perhaps she did not realise how much these women had suffereded, and how they deserved some part of the compensation that was being suggested by the government? Since 1989, the Medical Council had asked successive health ministers to introduce legislation giving the council new powers to act against doctors who placed people's lives or health in danger. Despite repeated promises, for well over a decade the Department of Health has failed to produce this vital legislation. Of course the question must also be asked as to why the Medical Council was urgently seeking this legislation? What knowledge did they have of poor medical skills in Ireland that was alarming them? Dr Tony Humphries, a clinical psychologist, aptly wrote in 2010:

> Is there a culture in Ireland that medical professionals are above the law? In the case of Michael Neary, the government has made no attempt to bring a legal case against him. Dr Neary's behaviour certainly had deep and disturbing unconscious sources. But whatever the neglect he experienced as a child, as an adult he is accountable for his actions and also accountable for seeking help with 'his issues'.

What a shame that clinical psychologists like Dr Humphries are not employed to care for doctors' mental and emotional health and well-being. Surely such care should be paramount, since doctors are on the front line, facing illness and death every day. In Ireland many young men and women study medicine. But this does not necessarily mean that they tolerate illness and death better than anyone else, or that all of them have the compassion needed to make good doctors. They too need ongoing guidance and counselling.

I have long held the view that if highly competent psychologists such as Dr Humphries had clinical access to Dr Neary, he might not have caused so much destruction and butchery. His predilection for removing wombs might have been discovered and controlled. While that possibility comes too late for many us, it could, if instituted, have the benefit of saving men and women from expressing such traumas in the future. Dr Humphries continued:

> The reluctance to pursue medical professionals for neglect of service users has echoes of the conspiracy between state and church in the cover-ups of the sexual abuse of children in the past.
>
> There has been a cleverly designed assumption that education brings maturity, but the facts do not support this claim. If politicians want to demonstrate eligibility to govern, let them first take the sty out of their own eyes and practise mature responses to uncovered neglects – wherever they occur.

Other theorists state that Neary had a morbid fear of haemorrhage: a fear or a phobia – who knows? If he did suffer this fear, he should have been man enough to seek professional help. No one is beyond getting sick or needing help, and yet there seems to be an assumption out there that we are not entitled to suffer human frailty. Such a fear on Neary's behalf was extremely harmful to many mothers. It is equally incomprehensible that any doctor with such a fear of blood would remain in the profession, especially as a surgeon. This is more ludicrous when that person chooses to work in obstetrics and gynaecology. Women bleed as an integral part of their femininity. But following childbirth, women are at their bloodiest, so any doctor suffering from a phobia of blood would surely feel tortured.

One wonders how such a previously busy man can now content himself with so much time on his hands and such a heavy conscience. Above all, he is human, and as such must feel the pressures that have been piled upon him, albeit largely of his own making. Some say he attends Mass, so it is unclear whether he has had some crisis of conscience. But he and I have the same maker, so it is not for me to judge.

With the likely state of Neary's inner confusion, I would not be surprised if he felt like he was the victim in all of this. He believed that someone was out to get him. Commenting on the mysterious removal of files, he said it was done by someone with an agenda to harm him. Again, then, I ask, what was it is all about? Justine McCarthy wrote in the *Irish Independent* in 2006 that:

He was a psychological cocktail of rampant egotism and professional ineptitude. But, amazingly, there are still those who swear by him. There is no unanimity of opinion about Michael Neary. Those who suffered at this surgeon's hands would be saints to ever forgive him, but there is sympathy for him among his more fortunate patients.

Neary has never been criminally charged, nor served a single day in prison. The worst he suffered was being struck off the medical register to practice by the Medical Council in 2003, having being found guilty of professional misconduct.

It smacks of the idea that white-collar crime pays. He achieved and still receives a sizeable pension, but no punishment for his misdeeds. Bad bankers, bad doctors, bad civil servants, bad company directors all seem to get rewarded with hefty pensions, severance pay and, often, a bonus to boot. Is it a case of the bigger the crime, the better the pension?

Yet, if an unemployed individual is caught doing a 'nixer' to subsidise his family's income, he probably loses his unemployment benefit, often has to face a court case and possibly even imprisonment. While I am in no way condoning fraudulent behaviour, there is a blatant disparity here.

So perhaps my solicitor was correct: nobody had ever taken a case against a doctor in Ireland, because they would have been fighting a 'system'. There was an obvious hierarchical culture pertaining at that time, which I think still exists.

Doctors were respected like God. Nobody questioned them, and they were regarded as superior to everybody else. It was almost a culture of fearful respect. This was my experience as a student at the hospital from 1975 to 1979. We were taught that the consultants employed at that time were the four pillars of the Lourdes Hospital, along with the MMMs. There was a clear inference that we owed them a debt of gratitude, and that they were above reproach. I often felt that even the MMM nursing sisters were afraid to question these men, and that they almost constantly felt subservient to them.

In seeking to prove that their hysterectomies were unnecessary, many women opted for Dr Roger Clements, a British consultant, to review their charts. He did not agree with the benign assessment which suggested that Neary had a phobia or fear of blood loss. Instead, he asked how Neary could explain the other separate gynaecological procedures that resulted in missing ovaries in sixty-two women? These women were, after all, neither bleeding from childbirth nor at death's door, as he had claimed that so many of his victims were. In order to justify the removal of their ovaries, these patients were told that they had endometriosis or cancer. According to Dr Clements the majority of these women did not suffer from either condition. Why would anyone want to play the role of Dr Death? It is beyond belief that anybody would instil such unnecessary fear, especially a doctor, in a vulnerable woman. Not only were they now grieving for the loss of their womb, but they were also made fearful by being given a groundless cancer diagnosis. These women were not included in the inquiry or redress schemes for compensation until much later, and following immense pressure. Later, after an investigation commissioned by Patient Focus, Dr Clements stated:

These weren't mistakes, they weren't carelessness; he, for some reason, had to perform these operations, and I can't understand the motivation. Neary exaggerated difficulties in the surgeries in order to convince those around him or those looking at the notes afterwards that he was justified in his surgery, but that clearly was not the case. I believe that Judge Harding Clark was too gentle on him.

Many changes have been recommended, and I hope that lessons can be learned from the Neary revelations and subsequent inquiries. One can only wonder if these recommendations have been fully implemented and are now part of daily practice at the Lourdes Hospital. Hopefully, with the recommendations that have now been made, some future good can come out of badness of the Neary inquest. It is an inescapable conclusion, from the many reports made into maternity practices at the Lourdes Hospital, that the obstetric profession has been exposed as having dangerous deficiencies. This is further evidenced in another separate investigation of symphysiotomy, which I will soon explain. Here, once again, it appears that the Lourdes Hospital operated this barbaric practice long after the rest of the country had opted against it.

Meanwhile, obstetricians were being treated with compassion and collegiality. It could not be thought of as unreasonable rubbish that intending parents might justifiably ask how safe our Irish maternity units are today. Many parents-to-be are filled with trepidation at the prospect of having to enter such units because of their well-publicised legacies. Unfortunately, until we have an independent and transparent mechanism for regulating obstetricians and maternity hospitals, we will never know the truth or full extent of what is currently going on in this field. We need an independent eagle eye to watch over the system and report appropriately for the sake of patient safety.

Personally, I continue to feel disbelieved by the medical

profession and the government in my quest for justice. How long do I have to wait to get that admission of wrongdoing, and an apology for being purposefully maimed? It may take thirty years, by which point the information can be disclosed under the Freedom of Information Act. Because of the mentality that prevailed in 1995 and beyond, I feel that my situation was minimised by all who looked at my notes, and misread the truth. Consequently, I got no opportunity to re-visit decisions made on my failed redress application. Above all, I feel that my perinatal hysterectomy was performed as an unjust means of sterilisation, without my knowledge and against my will. With hindsight, this belief is surely confirmed on my return postnatal visit when Neary said: 'At least now you can have free sex.' That statement seems weighted with intent.

As the late Gerry Conlon of the Guildford Four said on his release from wrongful imprisonment: 'There has been a serious miscarriage of justice.' It took many years for him to receive an admission of wrongdoing and a public apology from the relevant authorities. I believe that his traumatic experiences eventually led to his early demise.

We mothers have also suffered a serious miscarriage of justice, but no such apology is forthcoming. Perhaps they are waiting for our demise, too.

It no longer really matters to me what those in power think, promise but do not deliver, say or have said or how they have coloured the truth; they will have to live with their own consciences. I am a strong advocate for justice. It is what is in your heart and soul that is relevant; that is where the truth lies.

For those of you who have been injured by Neary or otherwise affected by medical negligence, please allow me to share an insight which I have found helpful in my personal recovery.

When you justifiably feel hurt as a result of your injury, you are faced with only two choices. You can lie down under it and waste the rest of your life as it takes you over like a cancer. In this approach, *you* are the only person still being hurt, while the perpetrators have long forgotten your circumstances. As we know, we have a relatively short span on this earth, so it would be a double tragedy to waste that precious time in continuing suffering and misery.

Alternatively, you can rise above it and make a new, albeit different beginning. In no way am I assuming this will be easy: there may be many obstacles and setbacks along the way, but you must never give up. After all, what is your real alternative? A friend once said to me in my time of need, 'If life gets too hard to stand, then kneel and crawl until you feel you can stand again.' The lesson in this is that we all have to start with mini-steps.

There are really good professionals out there who have a moral conscience, and can help you through this. Surround yourself with loving family members and friends who care deeply for you and you will not only survive, you will win and recover. We must embrace pain and burn it as fuel for our journey. This advice is in no way meant as condescension or to undermine or minimise what you are going through. Remember, I am one of you too, and this is how I have attempted to rise again. Neither is this an instruction to avoid pursuing these people through the legal system if those channels are still open to you.

If you have had a hysterectomy and are left without any children, or fewer than you would wish for, then that is a real travesty which nothing I will say can heal. But in rising above this, difficult as it may be, ask what God's plan is for your life, what is it He really wants from you and for you. What is your mission as laid out by him, because you matter to God. You also do not have to give birth biologically to give life: you can also give life by enhancing the lot of those more deprived, who, without your assistance, may never have survived. So often have I seen this with couples who adopted or fostered children as a result of their own misfortunes, thus giving life to children otherwise condemned to the loneliness of living in institutions.

Neither Dr Neary nor the hospital has ever accepted responsibility for the removal of women's wombs. In one case, it was reported that Neary's comment to a mother, when he informed her he had performed a hysterectomy, was: 'I took the cradle and left the playpen.' This is not the language of a normal, compassionate person, much less a doctor. I wonder if he even privately knew what he did was wrong? What he did was tantamount to abuse.

★

In 2010, Prime Time were doing a documentary for RTÉ on symphysiotomy. When caught on camera by the RTÉ investigators, Neary was asked about the women who had symphysiotomy performed. He simply said: 'I think these women just smell money.' This does not sound like a remorseful man. This does not sound like a doctor.

Symphysiotomy is a surgical procedure first advocated in 1597, in which the cartilage attached to the pubic symphysis bone was cut or divided to widen the pelvis in obstructed labour. It was done to allow childbirth if there was a mechanical problem, and when there was no option of performing a caesarean section. This procedure went into decline in the Western world in the late nineteenth century, when caesarean sections became the preferred option, though it is still performed when caesarean section is not an option. There was a brutality against women in this procedure, as many suffered immeasurably in the aftermath, and were left disabled for life. There were high associated risks, including urethral and bladder injury, infection, ongoing pain and long-term walking difficulties.

In the Republic of Ireland, however, an estimated 1,500 women unknowingly and without consent underwent symphysiotomies during childbirth between 1944 and 1984. The RTÉ *Prime Time* documentary rocked many people to their core. It revealed that doctors performed this procedure in Ireland to ensure childbirth without limitation and to train medical personnel and perfect the surgery for Africa.

Survivors of Symphysiotomy was a representative group established in Ireland in 2002. Following the *Prime Time* documentary, Minister for Health Mary Harney was asked to initiate an independent inquiry. Instead, she commissioned the Institute of Obstetricians and Gynaecologists to inquire into itself, by reviewing operations carried out by some of its own members for teaching purposes. It is unbelievable that this was her response, given the nature of the previous scandals.

In March 2012, a successful case was taken to the High Court by a symphysiotomy sufferer, with a financial award being duly made. In June 2012, Professor Oonagh Walsh of University College Cork found that, while this procedure had been phased out in most obstetric institutions for several years, Our Lady of Lourdes Hospital, Drogheda, continued to practise the procedure until the early 1980s. One wonders why they were not keeping up with continuous professional development, leaving obstetricians unaware of the demise of such practices elsewhere.

In April 2013, following a Dáil debate on the matter, a bill was unanimously supported by the Dáil, to lift the statute of limitation for a period of one year, to enable all survivors to bring their cases to the Irish courts. In November 2013, Minister for Health Dr James Reilly announced that Judge Yvonne Murphy had been appointed to review the Professor Walsh report, and to meet with survivors, hospital authorities and insurers with a view to deciding on whether an ex gratia redress scheme would be preferred to allowing legal actions to proceed. The terms of reference for Judge Murphy's inquiry were widely criticised, and seen as an obstacle to allowing women to pursue court action. Additionally, the government no longer supported the statute of limitations bill adopted in April 2013.

In March 2014, the Survivors of Symphysiotomy group complained to the United Nations, claiming that the Irish State had violated the United Nations Convention against torture by failing to properly, thoroughly or impartially investigate the practice of symphysiotomy in Ireland. Under international law, victims have a right to an effective remedy. They felt that all the government envisaged for survivors was an ex gratia scheme that was based on no admission of wrongdoing.

Consequently, Ireland was examined by the United Nations Human Rights Committee in August 2014. The committee told the Irish authorities that it should open a prompt, independent and thorough investigation into cases of symphysiotomy. They continued: 'Ireland should also identify, prosecute and punish – where still possible – the perpetrators for performing symphysiotomy without patient consent. The remedy should include fair and adequate compensation and rehabilitation on an individual basis.' This will make for interesting reading when it happens. Many of the obstetricians responsible are since deceased, but not all. This can only serve as a further indictment on past obstetric practices in Ireland.

With all the scandals that have been recorded, a lot of public trust and respect has been lost by the medical profession. This is worsened when high-ranking doctors decide that a colleague's career is more important than the truth, more important than people's lives. There seems to be a culture, in Ireland, that medical professionals are above the law. 'First do no harm' is the oath that doctors swear to, and it is still applicable to their practice.

I am well aware that there are many excellent, upstanding doctors and medical staff, but scandals have a strange way of tarnishing everyone with the same brush. We must learn to segregate these, as good does prevail more often than evil within the profession, if we just choose to see it.

The Irish State, the government, still face many unanswered questions from its women. To say that Ireland is at last 'facing up to its murky past' in relation to women is nonsense, as with each new scandal we hear similar rhetoric being trotted out: 'This must never be allowed to happen again.' Such announcements often mistakenly and falsely gives an impression to the public that these women have all been compensated. Is it not the State's responsibility to ensure that patients are properly protected from negligent medical staff and, where negligence does occur, that the injured are duly compensated? Instead, there are only penny-pinching compensation measures given eventually – if at all – while the legal teams scoop up the Irish taxpayers' lottery. During my training we repeatedly listened to Neary talk about the high cost of his professional insurance. Why then were his insurers not compelled to pay for his negligence, rather than the taxpayers?

Despite repeated requests from the Medical Council since 1989, successive health ministers have failed to introduce legislation against doctors who placed people's lives at risk. This has been despite some shocking scandals which should have set off alarm bells. These have included the adults who died at the hands of Dr Harold Shipman in Great Britain, the deaths of children at the Bristol Royal Infirmary and others. Yet, the Irish government made no attempt to bring a criminal case against Neary for the mayhem he caused. It is as if they have turned a blind eye. This echoes the strong sense of fear there seems to have been in regard to challenging Church members. The Church-versus-State fiscal responsibility was not the strong suit of theprevailing government. We all remember when Minister Woods, on the eve of a general election, managed to sign a child abuse deal allowing the Catholic Church to pay only 10 percent of the child-abuse bill. Are votes and individual TDs seats more important than injured people?

The government of the day were also negligent in not including all women injured by Neary in the redress scheme. Women suffered immensely, and continue to suffer, as a result of what happened. Women are still being disbelieved. Their suffering includes the financial loss either from not being able to work, and/or the financial outlay incurred in attempting to recover some sense of normality. While the current government has made some attempts to address this, there is much, much more to be done to defray this loss.

If politicians are serious about their duty to govern, then they need to take the plank out of their eye and practise some mature responses to the uncovered neglects, whatever they may be. I do not appreciate opposition politicians making political mileage out of our tragedies; this is a recipe for further disasters and serves only as an insult to the women involved.

The complex nature of abuse is a minefield. Sadly, our Irish history has recorded a major disrespect for women. We have had the Magdalene Laundries scandal, which demonised women, and took years for any shred of wrongdoing to be acknowledged, until Taoiseach Enda Kenny did so. This government has gone some way down that road, for which I am sure the women are grateful. They received an apology, which was huge. But, for many of them, it is too little too late. And have they actually received their compensation? Those affected by symphysiotomy are still in a wilderness, wondering what shape their redress will take following the European directive.

Now we are faced with the mother and baby homes scandal. Once again, women are demonised. The sad fact here is that these unmarried women were branded harlots. But where were the fathers responsible for these pregnancies? Why were they never sought, demonised and made to pay restitution? Many of these women hardly knew the facts of life, much less what was happening to their bodies when they were pregnant. When I worked in a geriatric hospital, many of the elderly women recounted these stories to me. Their tales would have broken the hardest heart. I know of many women who were incarcerated in psychiatric hospitals as a consequence of being unmarried mothers, many remaining in these institutions for the remainder of their lives. They were abandoned by their families, often due to poverty and shame, and rarely received visitors. Thrown onto the scrapheap of life, they were forgotten about. We are told that all babies are a gift from God. Why then did religious communities treat these unfortunate women with such disdain, cruelty and hardship?

On the other hand, without the religious orders taking these women in, there was often nowhere for them to go, as the State at that time provided no alternate accommodation for them and their babies. It bears a stark resemblance to Mary and Joseph on the imminent birth of Jesus.

We still repeatedly hear of women having hysterectomies, whether perinatal or otherwise. Little remarks like this are passed on, and it is viewed as acceptable. But if a man must suffer from the removal of a genital organ it is thought of as shocking. It is treated very differently, and taken much more seriously. Why is this?

In the past, my anger was open and apparent, but, over time and with much help, I have tried to let it go in my decision to rise above it and daily strive to get my life back, albeit in a different fashion. Life is finite, and only God knows how much time any of us have left. My husband, my children and my parents were my greatest 'landing pad', my support. They deserve an Oscar for what they have tirelessly done. Close friends and colleagues were wonderful, during those years – towers of strength.

Many of the therapists and therapies helped, to some extent. But for me, I have found that cognitive behaviour therapy finally 'cracked it'. This therapy is helping me to drop my emotional baggage piece by piece, and let go of old negative feelings that were haunting me; it is making me realise that the only person hurting is me.

It was as if I was on a cobbled path that often did not make sense, but that has inched me along the way to recovery. Of course, I still have my bad, black days where I feel everything all over again.

Panic attacks are never too far away much of the time, but the difference is that now I realise that these attacks will not kill me. Simple techniques like my daily thankfulness list, exercise and my 'breakfast with God' help me keep going. I move on however, with an indelible mark, and with my life having changed negatively in so many ways. Exercise is an amazing tonic in this state. We must continue to push ourselves out of our comfort zones, and try 2 percent harder. It does pay off.

'Anger is an acid that can do more harm to the vessel in which it is stored than to anything on which it is poured'
                                                            –Mark Twain

So why should I hold on to anger?

Life has changed, not ended. Life's legacy should be greater than one's lifespan. I feel that the only place where success comes before work is in the dictionary. I work daily to improve my lot, as I do not want my obituary to read, 'What might have been.'

As long as I am still breathing, I can close the gap between what is and what can or might have been. My biggest tool for renewal has been, and continues to be, my faith. I thank my parents for handing me such a wonderful tool. While I have 'let rip' at God, often wondering if he even existed, bargaining with and badgering Him, I am grateful for having the faith to realise that life is a vale of tears. What I have gone through is like a death. Everybody gets crosses in life to bear, some seemingly greater than others, but, as they say, God fits the back for the burden.

Much blame has been attributed to the Catholic Church in this scandal and others cited heretofore. But we need to draw a distinction between the Catholic Church and those who operate within it: its members, those who call themselves Catholics. The Catholic Church has clearly laid down certain teachings that some who operate within it have chosen to break. For me, Neary broke those rules, not the Church. So, is the Catholic Church really responsible? Given all the scandals I have cited, if Jesus was the manager in charge of any of these situations I feel sure he would have done many things differently.

In his evidence to the Harding Clark Inquiry, Neary recounted being summoned to a meeting by the late Cardinal Ó Fiach, Archbishop of Armagh, who, as a result of his was patron of the Lourdes Hospital. In that statement, Neary said that the Cardinal threatened, that, if he broke the hospital's code of ethics, he would ensure that his brother would lose his teaching job in Cork. I question why such threats were made, and actual disciplines not imposed.

Do I forgive Dr Neary? Yes, I forgive the man, because it helps me to continue with my life. But I am absolutely entitled to challenge his behaviour and the hurt inflicted on me personally and on my family.

My situation took place during an era when Church teaching was, as Justice Harding Clark stated, 'caught in a time warp'. But Neary still had no right to do what he wanted for his own personal vindication or heroism, rather than what the patients needed or agreed to. Time warp or not, we were not given a second chance, so why was he?

The Harding Clark Inquiry concluded that he probably panicked on a regular basis over his twenty-five-year career. Dr Maresh did not accept this. I know all too well what that feels like, but I do not injure people as a result of my panic. Rather, I chose to seek help. Was he too proud to seek that help, or curtail his practice until he felt better or had sorted out his feelings?

Professionals often are not asked to make themselves accountable for their own behaviour. Much of this is due to a lack of auditing of their performance. But, in my opinion, Neary needs to examine his conscience in regards to his professional performance.

We are all given a conscience and a soul. Each of us needs to regularly examine our own conscience and soul. Dr Barry taught me that we are all 'raggy dolls': that we have all messed up several times during our lives. But we must strive to do better. We must forgive ourselves and others each day that we live and, above all, we must not harm others in the process.

I am well aware that many of you mothers are still hurting, many in silence. We all face crises in our lives in very different ways. Those who took part in this castration process abused women and tore at the very fabric of our society, denying the opportunity to those future generations to make any impact, denying you the knowledge of what impact your children might have had on our nation.

Yes, I am starkly aware that our wombs cannot be replaced, that the chance of giving birth has been taken away forever. Time is not a healer, it simply helps you accept living with your loss, but there is always an indelible mark left. Many of us have been castigated by those regarded as 'important professional reviewing consultants', but never allow them to take your spirit.

You matter.

I said at the outset that, in this book, I would outline my experience, and that is what I have done. I know the facts of what happened to me, and only I can stand over my experience.

Chapter 17
I Only Went in to Have My Baby

'At last I have cast away the old that I might now be free,
At last I'm graced to see the things I have always yearned to see.
At last I am becoming the woman I have always longed to be.
And that's the woman who is never alone,
And that woman, at last, is me.'

–'The Cradle of Eternity'

In life there is nothing more important than to show each person that they are unique, that they have a purpose, that they are of value to society, and that they matter. For many of us mothers, our experience at the hands of Dr Neary was far from showing us that we matter.

We must nevertheless aspire to mental fitness, as this is vital to our future recovery. This is necessary for our survival, despite constant uncertainty and change in our lives from our past experiences. Otherwise, we roller-coaster up and down the scale of happiness, constantly falling back into the cocoon of our unique comfort zone, whatever form that may take. While our comfort zone is important, as it is where we feel safe, it does not allow us to grow and progress, and can close in around us if we are not watchful, overpowering us if we are not careful. This, if we allow it to, can ultimately leave us sitting on the edge of our seats much of the time, in a state of impending panic. We must gradually appreciate ourselves, our self-worth and our self-esteem in a habit-forming manner. Learn to put yourself in your diary today, and be consistent and resilient in this habit. But be mindful of being gentle with yourself, and grit your teeth as you make that 2 percent change daily. There will of course be days when you scale right back down, but climb again as you must and as you can. Any person, particularly a doctor, who chooses to abuse women by mutilating their bodies to prevent them from having children, tears at the core fabric of our society and our nation. This vandalising behaviour must never be acceptable, in any society. Irrespective of prevailing circumstances, 'time warp' and regimes at the time, irrespective of Neary's personal viewpoint on Church teaching, *nobody* gave him permission to inflict such abuse and harm.

Nobody gave him free rein to attain his personal agenda. If he suffered from panic, or blood phobia, or felt incompetent, then it was his personal responsibility to ask for help, to ask for a second opinion from colleagues – even to stop practising. None of us are above making mistakes, or are big to ask for help. We are, after all, all 'raggy dolls'.

Life has thrown me some curve balls which were not always easily borne. Even in the midst of suffering at the hands of Neary, even with the grave miscarriage of justice doled out to me, life goes on with all its challenges, and time does not stand still. My children have pretty much grown up now, and are moving to new phases in their own lives. Unfortunately, life does not pause or wait for you to get well.

I still thank God that he chose me to bear these crosses rather than my children. I am fortunate to have six beautiful, wonderfully gifted children, and one angel. I often worried about my capability as a mother, since I was suffering from post-traumatic stress, and felt inadequate. They have never brought the police to my door, never been culprits of the social vices of today and, for that, I am eternally grateful. Arlene's nomination of me for the Mother of the Year award eased many of those fears, and I am eternally grateful for it. I feel so humbled by her nomination and the gratitude and insight shown by my children in appreciating their mother. Being the eldest, she in many ways assumed my role in the family for many years, along, indeed, with the others. I was amazed, honoured and humbled when I was crowned Ulster Mother of the Year 2012. Above all else, it taught me that I must have done something right, and that my children cherished me for the good and through the suffering – that is what this award really meant to me, nothing more prestigious than that. I pray that it has taught them that suffering is an integral part of life. Ironically, when a friend phoned me the next day to congratulate me, she asked if I was still on 'cloud nine'. My answer was the truth: 'I am on my knees as we speak, scrubbing a floor.' My roots have taught me well to stay grounded.

I am grateful for the many true friends, fabulous colleagues and, above all else, the family members who have picked me up along the way. I am also eternally grateful for those who encouraged me to keep a journal and write this book. You are true masters ofdestiny, and strong swords in my recovery.

I hope this book will resonate with many of you for a variety of reasons. I also hope it has given you the confidence to pick up the fragile pieces of your life and recover whatever fragments you can while there is still time.

My wish is that it gives you hope and confidence to:

- Know that how you are feeling is not always your fault.

- Speak out when you have a cause to champion.

- Move forward, even in mini-steps, but do take that first step; remember that 2 percent change can make 100 percent difference.

- Respect life with all your being: suicide is never an answer, as it simply adds more misery to those who really, genuinely love you.

- Recover well and remember that each new day is God's gift to you, and what you do with it is your gift to God.

- Accept that you are enough, you don't need to be anything that you are not.

From my work of thirty years as a practitioner in my clinic, I realise that many people have a surprising amount of emotional trauma in their energy fields, which lie below their conscious awareness, in a core place of restriction, stored in their sub- conscious mind. The core place of this constriction can block the life force within, leading to the ill effects of physical or mental disease, or both at the more serious end of the spectrum. Illness can start as an emotion. If it is not properly dealt with and healed, then it will ultimately manifest as a physical illness, its range of effect, dependent on the core trauma.

I have seen mothers who have lost a child develop breast cancer. I have seen people suffering from unresolved grief, a fear of speaking up for themselves or not being listened to or being heard, develop progressive lung problems. I have seen people who can't cope with the 'nonsense' in their life develop bowel cancer. I have seen women whose female side has been immensely hurt suffering from uterine, ovarian or breast problems.

Unconsciously, we can perfect the denial of emotional pain in an attempt to function daily, to survive in a false sense of un-reality. It is as if we are keeping the pain at bay, but for how long? This creates such internal imbalance that it becomes distorted. Our only sense of this is feeling 'off' within, and looking for external answers to fix us. It is at this point that we may develop our 'ism'. To 'fix' ourselves we need to look further within for the cause. I believe this can be attained through proper therapy, but is not always well served by medication alone. Only then can the real being within ourselves be revealed.

At the core of this is a belief or thought that we are not good enough, or that we have done something wrong. This generally comes from rocking the boat of a caregiver, which unconsciously triggers their unhealed wounds from their past, and their action gets projected onto the caregiver.

Some of us have been emotionally frozen out from our feelings. We innately know that something is wrong, but the feelings them-selves become indefinable. This is an action from that part of us to protect us from the intolerable pain and shame of powerlessness that we feel if we think we are bad at a core level. We need to give ourselves permission to feel the fear within, in order to start healing. True, we can never change what has happened to us, but we can initiate change in how we are coping – or not. This allows us to move forward. Forgiveness is not tantamount to condoning the action, the person or the situation, but a lack of forgiveness serves only to keep us holding onto a deep sense of rejection and betrayal. As previously stated, anger is like an acid that does more harm to the vessel it is contained in than anything it can be poured on. Progressively, this can cause disease: that is, the body is not at ease with itself, which in turn can cause deeper and more serious illness. Hospitals or other institutions cannot do that healing for you; you must be ready to try to heal within yourself. Your cognitive understanding and your gut instinct must be in tandem. Of course, not all of us make a full recovery, or even a partial recovery. It would be romantic to think we will all sail into the sunset as very happy people, as if we were living life as a movie. Life is not a movie; this is the real deal, this is all we have. The truth is that we can move, but we remain scarred, each living our individual private dilemmas daily.

I speak from personal experience here. I have also seen this transition in so many people attending my clinic who did not believe or want to believe they were stressed to begin with until they faced their demons, and only then fully recovered their health.

In life, we all come up against rejection on many occasions, and in varying circumstances. I have felt rejected, an outcast, a leper, by many of those directed to help me during this crisis. These included some, but not all, doctors; the minister for health, in how she and her predecessor established the redress board and how she ignored my correspondence; the Lourdes Hospital, for not ensuring a place of safety to deliver my baby; the system – whatever that is.

I feel sure that many more women who have had a similar experience with Neary, or indeed comparable experiences in the wider medical field, have felt rejection and other feelings akin to mine, making each of you feel very insignificant, both fearful and tearful, and a whole mixed bag of other emotions.

Well, when God gives you a passion, when you are really set on making positive change, never feel that you are at a dead end. Do not be put off by rejection when your very soul tells you that you are working in the cause of right. Let me share a thought with you for where you are now: there comes a time in your life when you walk away from all the trauma, the drama and the people who created it. You surround yourself with people who make you laugh. Try to forget the bad, focus instead on the good in your life. If you cannot do that yet, then offer it up to the higher power, asking for His help. Love the people who treat you right, and pray daily for those who don't. Life is too short to be anything but happy; no day is worth living twice. Falling down is part of life; getting back up is called living.

You may not be there yet, but keep going – you can win. You may be one of those women who has never had the opportunity to be a mother, or a mother who has had her future biological opportunities surgically taken away from her. Nothing can change that, unfortunately.

Please look into your heart and ask what God and the universe are asking of you and have in store for you, because they most likely have carved out another niche for you in life. Your destiny, your role may be as a great mother figure, a life-saver to others.

I do not know the identity of the midwives who were the whistleblowers, or their whereabouts. But as a woman, a mother and a survivor, I wish to thank you, the midwives, for your bravery, your moral courage to stand up in the cause of right – your tenacity. Sadly, your bravery came too late for me and many other women. But rest assured that you have saved many other mothers from the clutches of such a surgical predator. I have no doubt you felt vilified by your actions. This came from many sources I'm sure, some very unexpected.

Let me also extend that thanks to those in the North-Eastern Health Board who listened to me and heard me. Without their subsequent actions, the midwives' concerns would have fallen on deaf ears.

As student nurses we were taught by the Medical Missionaries of Mary that we must live within our moral code, trust our gut instinct and not participate in what goes against our religion. That we must have the moral courage to walk away if we see a procedure that we cannot participate in, and at all times be true to ourselves. That was wise teaching, but obviously not widely heeded by many. When one tries to speak out, the reactions may be very different, but right is right even if no one else is doing it and wrong is wrong even if everyone else is doing it. Let negative reaction never stop you or discourage you. Stand alone and be brave if necessary.

So, keep going in the name of good, justice and right. Do not pray for a lighter burden, instead pray for a stronger back to carry it. Try to put your past behind you and begin again, because change is the essence of life. Attempt to look for something positive in each day, even if some days you have to look a little harder.

It has taken me nineteen years to get to a better place, and this still remains a daily challenge. That has taken a lot of perseverance, a lot of therapy and a huge financial cost for which I have never been reimbursed. Writing this book, for me, has been hugely cathartic, therapeutic and healing. I wish to stand up and be a voice for the voiceless. I alone cannot change the world, but by casting a stone into the waters I can make many ripples. I can now say I forgive Dr Michael Neary but not his behaviour, and I wish him all the luck he deserves. After all, we will both have to meet our maker some day. Forgiveness is not condoning the action of the perpetrator, and a lack of forgiveness prevents one from moving forward. For those of you who have been injured in life by this man or others, I hope that my closing wish will lend a little comfort to you.

Today, may you experience peace within.

May you trust that you are exactly where you are meant to be.

May you not forget the infinite possibilities that are born of faith in yourself and others.

May you use the gifts that you have received throughout your life, and pass on the love that has been given to you.

May you be content with yourself just the way you are.

Let this knowledge settle into your bones, and allow your soul the freedom to sing, dance, praise and love. It is there for each and every one of us.

As C.S. Lewis said: 'You are never too old to set another goal or to dream a new dream.'

I have given many valuable years to monstrous turmoil, but

now I have turned the corner, and so can you. No matter what our circumstances, we always have something to be thankful for. Be who you are, and be well.

I wish you love and light in your quest for recovery and enlightenment.

Yours for good health,
Kathleen

Appendix A

A VIOLATION AGAINST WOMEN

Dr. ███████ MD, FRCOG
Consultant Obstetrician and Gynaecologist

OUR LADY OF LOURDES HOSPITAL,
DROGHEDA, CO. LOUTH.
Tel. 041-983 7601
Fax 041-987 4762

SHEELIN, NORTH ROAD,
DROGHEDA, CO. LOUTH.
Tel. 041-987 3525
Fax 041-980 4217

10th July 2015

Ms. Kathleen Ward
████████████

CO. MONAGHAN

Dear Kathleen,

Please find enclosed a copy of your notes and correspondence from your consultation
with me in 1999 . If there is anything else you require please request this is writing.

Trusting this finds you well.

Yours sincerely,

███████ MD., FRCOG
Consultant Obstetrician & Gynaecologist

KATHLEEN WARD

6ᵗʰ December 1999

Dr. ███████

███████

CO. MONAGHAN

RE: **Kathleen Ward**
███████████████████████████, **Monaghan**

     DOB: 28/05/56

Dear Dr. ████

Thank you for sending along this nice lady with her interesting history. Her symptoms would certainly fit in with Menopausal Status.

I see Dr. Neary's note that her Ovaries were conserved at the time of Hysterectomy, but as with her recent Ultrasound, I can see no evidence of these on Scan again today. However, there is quite an amount of Uterus still left in situ. This would indeed explain all her problems and by the time you get this I will have spoken to you about her Hormone Profile, which you have checked.

Kathleen now realises that indeed that her Uterus was not ruptured and that the baby was not lying free in the Peritoneal Cavity as she was told by Dr. Neary and perhaps also her ovaries may have been taken in contrast as to what was noted. We will have to wait and see for now.

Yours sincerely,

███████████ MRCOG
Consultant Obstetrician & Gynaecologist